Cancer Looks Good on You

Cancer Looks Good on You

BARCLAY FRYERY
AND JILL JOHNSON

Barclay's Guide to Cultivating **Style,** Sanity,
Silliness and Self-Love—in Sickness and in Health

PARIS LION PRESS

Published 2017

Printed in the United States of America
Hardcover ISBN: 978-0-9990680-0-7
Paperback ISBN: 978-0-9990680-1-4
E-ISBN: 978-0-9990680-2-1
Library of Congress Control Number: 2017908775

Cover design by Yoonsun Lee and Tabitha Lahr
Interior design by Tabitha Lahr

For information, visit: CancerLooksGoodonYou.com

To Daniel,
For without Dr. Frankenstein,
there would be no Frankenstein.

"Nothing is impossible.
The word itself says "I'm possible!"
—AUDREY HEPBURN

Contents

Prologue

IN MAY OF 2016, BARCLAY FRYERY made a trip to Greenwich, Connecticut, from Meridian, Mississippi, his hometown. He had lived much of his aspirational adult life in Greenwich, surrounded by beauty—the lovely cafes and boutiques lining Greenwich Avenue, a pretty and pedigreed social set, his exquisite apartment (which was featured in *House Beautiful* and *Elle Decor*). For Barclay, life brimmed with possibility here: interior decorating for the rich and famous, a newspaper advice column, a TV show, a furniture line, a book project, evening soirees in Greenwich and nearby New York, lunches al fresco on warm spring days.

When we met at National Café on May 20, it was the beginning of sandal season. The sky had dressed in pure blue that morning. The promise of a summer tan lingered in the air. It was a dazzling day, a day for big dreams and grand designs. I saw Barclay striding down Greenwich Ave, dapper as always in a crisp white button-down shirt, with a navy sweater thrown over his shoulder and his signature dark sunglasses on. He still stood tall (hard not to at 6'6"), with more of a paunch than he had in his younger years, but that's to be expected at 55. I thought to myself, *Everything is going to be okay.*

Barclay saw me and gave me a hug that erased the gap of several years without seeing each other. He beamed that familiar smile, the one that can light up a ballroom or make a lowly cashier or busboy feel special (he bestowed one on the National Café hostess as well, before calling her by name and asking how she was doing; n*o one* is lowly in Barclay's eyes). We sat down at the table Barclay—always attending to aesthetic details—requested. I looked into his weary but eager eyes and said, "Cancer looks good on you, Barclay."

For two years Barclay had been waging war on this *ugly* disease, which had attacked his lymph nodes. He'd retreated to Mississippi to fight the battle among "his pretty things," which he'd transported from Greenwich, but also the scars from growing up as Timothy Mark Fryery, a closeted gay boy in the Deep South. He'd won that war, made a new name for himself—literally and figuratively—and led a life he never could have imagined was possible in his youth. Surely he could win this war too.

Now we sat enjoying our salads and recounting old times, when I was the editor of *Tear Sheet*, a magazine I launched in my wide-eyed twenties, and Barclay, in his decadent thirties, had reported on fashion and life from Paris for me. We became friends. Barclay oozes his own blend of *joie de vivre* and genuine charm that's irresistible.

We talked about radiation, the dark abysses along the way, and the hills he has climbed with his indomitable spirit, reaching a scenic overlook with a view onto a future dotted with more possibilities. He was excited to travel to the Bahamas to do Bill

Ford's wedding. Bill, son of Ford Model matriarch Eileen, would marry Barclay's dear friend Darrah Gleason Ford. He imagined moving back to Greenwich and continuing the career that earned him a coveted spot in *House Beautiful*'s Top 100 Designers list for a decade. He said he planned to travel to Greenwich again in the fall. We could do lunch again; he had some contacts who might help me with publishing my modeling memoir.

A DIFFERENT BOOK PROJECT altogether has emerged since then. As the posts on Barclay's Facebook page, where he blogs prolifically about his cancer journey, grew more earnest, I had a nagging feeling. It was easy to dismiss it because Barks, as I like to call him, always flashes plenty of bright thoughts into the darkness. He has an inner beacon of light that is impossible to snuff out.

But on March 10, 2017, Barclay shared a video of himself with his 10,000 Facebook followers. In a composed and calm manner, he announced: "Hi, it's Barclay. I promised you an update. I just returned from the hospital and the doctors have decided there is nothing more they can do, and I'm not going to do any more treatments. I'm just going to manage the symptoms with the pain doctor and with home health care, which will eventually become hospice. I'll be surrounded by my close friends and my animals and my pretty things. I don't want people to be upset, like a friend of mine has been all week. I love you. I've had so many people be nice to me and lovely to me." He paused here and his voice quavered as he continued more slowly, "I know it's hard to say this, but it's been a very nice period, even though it's been a bad period. And I just wanted to share that news with you."

The cancer had spread. The doctors gave my dear Barks two weeks to two months to live. His own best cancer cheerleader, Barclay did not dive off the top of the pyramid in dismay. He slowly dismounted and placed his rather swollen size-13 feet firmly on the ground. From there he would complete his final design project: the plans for a dignified, stylish, full final chapter on Earth and, of course, a fabulous after-party (both here, for the mortals, and in the afterlife).

THE GIFT AND THE CURSE OF CANCER is that you often know when the end is coming. You can say good-bye to friends. You can wrap up loose ends. You can dwell on death, fret, sweat, careen into depression. There will be none of that latter part for Barclay, at least not that he will reveal to the "angels" who care for him and the friends who come to visit him in his cozy and carefully curated apartment in downtown Meridian.

I booked my flight for a week after I saw Barclay's post. I didn't want to stall. I've been on one of these journeys before, when my grandmother lost her battle with stomach (and then bone) cancer. She was skeletal but lucid when I, at age 19, said good-bye. Entering the halls of a hospital always brings back that memory: the tender, heart-wrenching final embrace with my frail Grammie, amidst the harsh antiseptic smell and sterile furnishings of a 1980s hospital room. A week later she did not know anyone. Two weeks later she was gone.

In Barclay's Facebook posts, optimism continued to beat out suffering: "Good morning world!" or "Oo la la . . . Looking forward to a WONDERFUL DAY! Nothing will get in my way of having the best day possible!" Although there were some of these: "Having a horrific day. Please pray." I prayed he would keep his strength for many "wonderful" days to come, though I was sure it was a Barclay-ism (i.e., euphemism) for *bearable*. I braced myself for my visit.

I needn't have. My day with Barclay was inspiring, fascinating,

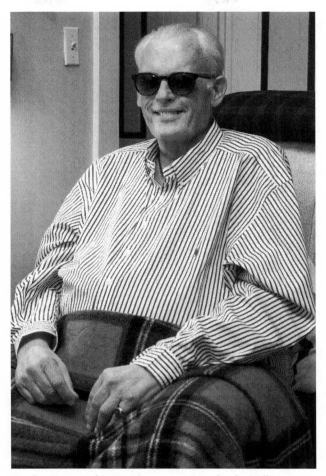

Barclay Fryery in his Meridian apartment, shot by William David Barr

warm, revelatory. I learned about his challenging childhood, his days in DC with the politicos, Paris and Greenwich with the fashion elite. How he handled a homophobic father, an HIV diagnosis, a cancer diagnosis. How he formed his brigade of angels who care for him now. I met two of them and learned how much he does for them in their visits, not just how much they do for him.

Susie Womack Cannon ("Choo" to Barclay, who is fond of

bestowing nicknames), his first babysitter and his first crush, explained it this way on Facebook: "It is Sunday morning and I am sitting here with Barclay enjoying his company. He is amazing, being determined to make something positive from all this. I'm one of three that have the privilege of caring for Barclay and he never ceases to amaze me in that we, who come to love on and encourage him, always leave feeling encouraged by him."

I talked by phone to his closest friend from his college years at Ole Miss. He shared funny stories about preppy Republican Barclay and his immaculate dorm room. I spoke to his friend Lauren in Greenwich, who has followed Barclay's fight with cancer on Facebook and calls him every single day. They have never met in person.

I recorded my eight-hour interview with Barclay because it was clear that Barclay has wisdom about *the end*—not to mention the beginning and the middle—that we all can learn from. This book is a gift from Barclay to you. It contains simple tips for infusing joy into a sorrowful time, deeper reflections on overcoming life's challenges, and a good dose of magical memories, too. Enjoy.

CHAPTER 1

Fluff

◦–◦–◦–◦–◦

Barclay's 5 Easy Ways to Take the Ugly Out of Sickly

READING THIS BOOK IS GOING TO be like peeling an onion. There will be some tears along the way, as each chapter delves deeper into a life and psyche that are much more complex than you might imagine. The lessons Barclay will impart in the process may be life-saving for readers—for victims of society's ills as much as for victims of disease. But we will start with the "fluff," the seemingly little things Barclay has done to take some of the ugly out of illness and infuse a dose of his signature style.

When Barclay descended into the trenches with cancer, when he really dug in and saw things getting grim, he felt compelled to settle into his homey apartment in Meridian and find solace. That is where I visit him today, not in a depressing hospital room like the one where I bid farewell to my grandmother.

As I arrived at the Georgian red brick four-plex where Barclay lives in a petite one-bedroom apartment, I noticed his pretty boxwood porch garden: classic terracotta mixed with raised panel French planters, an antique lantern beside a black wrought-iron chair, a black-and-white awning to shade the charming retreat from the scorching Mississippi sun. There was a touch of sophistication otherwise absent on the street I reached several turns after a store advertising "Beauty Supplies and School Uniforms" in huge bold letters.

The lovely Susie, a.k.a. "Choo," was attending to Barclay when I got there. Life has come full circle, since Susie was his first babysitter. Barclay is having a good day. He looks animated and his voice has all its usual richness and endearing Southern accent. "She was 11; I was 5. I had a huge crush on her," gushes Barclay. "I used to try to impress her doing tricks on my red tricycle. And now she is taking care of me. She is like an angel sent to me. We reconnected during cancer." (These reconnection and angel themes recur as the day goes on, and they will recur in this book as well.)

As Susie goes to leave, Barclay—who spends most of his day sitting, to rest his painfully swollen legs and feet—points to the pretty decorator pillows on the cushy chair (from the Barclay Fryery Collection) where I'm to sit. "Choo! You forgot to fluff that pillow!" he scolds with a chuckle. He's only half kidding. Barclay still takes pride in his surroundings. After all, his career was built on a perfectionist's attention to details like this.

Even for this average gal, whose design aesthetic has evolved little since college, the effect is that Barclay does not seem like someone who has given up. It does not feel like I am in a claustrophobic room with a friend who is dying and distraught. Even if he is both of those things, the very act of carrying on caring about the details makes him—and his parade of visitors—feel better about ugly reality.

Fluff Off, Cancer:
5 Easy Ways to Take the Ugly Out of Sickly

LESSON #1: BEAUTIFY YOUR SURROUNDINGS. Even when Barclay was relegated to a hospital room, he spurned the standard gowns in favor of his own clothing: freshly pressed Ralph Lauren button-down shirts, slim-cut jogging pants, Gucci loafers, and sunglasses. He brought throw pillows and his signature FDR Royal Stewart Tartan blanket to brighten up his room (he covers his legs with this blanket now, as we talk). His favorite teddy bear came along too. "I know it sounds silly," says Barclay, "but it made me happier." There are three on his bed at home, including one donning a fashionable scarf, and I'm sure he'd have a few words for anyone who feels too "old" for stuffed animals. He also uses designer pillows to serve the same purpose as a stodgy sleep apnea pillow. "I want to be hip," exclaims Barclay, "I don't want a hospital bed! Hospital beds, wheelchairs—no, no, no!" Barclay keeps a collection of antique walking canes by the front door; they are for decoration, not for the decrepit.

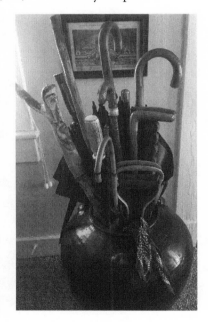

"I've pulled out the good towels, good linens, the real table napkins, and I use them, as opposed to hoarding them," adds Barclay. "I have so many things to look at that are pretty; it sounds vapid, but it helps get me through." His apartment does not have the sickening smell of an infirmary but rather a pleasing aroma of crisp white linen and lavender.

Barclay's bathroom features a silver tray, antique crystal decanters,

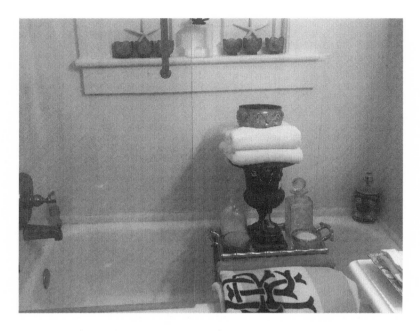

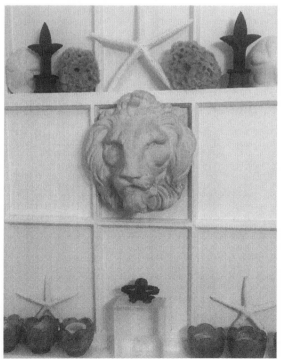

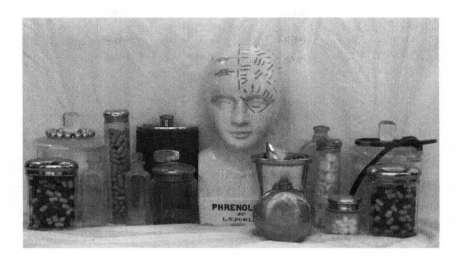

and an urn with fluffy white towels atop it—all in the tub. There are starfish to remind him of the seaside and a regal 19th-century lion mask because Barclay is a proud Leo (we agree that it is the very best sign). Most notably, a row of fitted sterling silver and crystal suitcase bottles filled with pills are lined up across the top of his vanity. "I brought back that idea from Pharmacy in London, a restaurant Damien Hirst did with a pill-oriented design. I thought, *Look, he's decorating with pills! I can too.*" The result is that the multifarious medications a cancer patient must take never looked so enticing.

With mounting medical bills, practicality has played a role in Barclay's design scheme. He has sold most of his modern paintings and good classic items. "I've kept just what I couldn't sell and mixed it up and made it work," he explains. "My books and portraits—that's the nutshell of my design here. The palette: I've used royal blue and punches of lipstick red and hot pink, mixed with natural colors." He hired a woman named Renae Gardner to do meticulous interior painting, including large elegant squares framing the ceilings. "They are inspired by the tents used during battle in Roman and Napoleonic times," explains Barclay.

"Banded tentings or togas were signs of great wealth. If you were going to die on the battlefield, you might as well go out in style. Hence the introduction of campaign style."

Now when Barclay is lying in bed, staring at the ceiling, it is not emptiness he sees . . . but a whole history of people determined to go out in style! He also sees the handiwork of someone who has become a dear friend. He and Renae now barter: his designer insider tips for her help caring for him. Beautifying leading to a beautiful friendship—who knew?

LESSON #2: SURROUND YOURSELF WITH HAPPY MEMORIES.
"I've edited table tops and moved things around," says Barclay of the visual feast in his space. "It's more cluttered than usual, but I wanted to be around as many pretty things as possible." His apartment, while busy in decor, is neat and tidy—another must to avoid a sense of things unraveling.

Barclay has added his favorite portraits of himself through the years to his walls: there is a painting of Barclay back when he was still "Timothy"; Barclay looking all *L'Uomo Vogue* in tweed in his 20s; Barclay at 32 and his first dog, a Puli named "Mr. Pooh," drawn by his artist friend Leslie Mueller; Barclay in black, eyes closed in meditation; and a rather famous painting of Barclay looking like a sexy mad scientist by Mary Newcomb.

Sentimental cards from friends are displayed on windowsills and Memento Boards—that's in caps because the boards are part of Barclay's furniture collection. "I designed them so you can post your memories and look at them when you are down, as opposed to a photo album you never open," says Barclay, who appreciates those boards now more than ever. Mixed with the cards are photos of family, friends, more than a few hunky men, and even modeling matriarch Eileen Ford out on the town in her twenties.

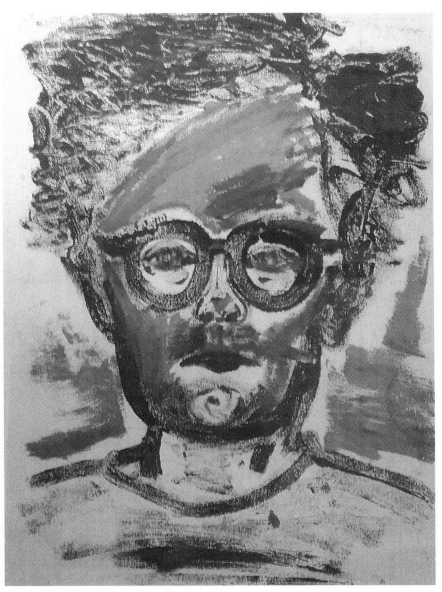

Barclay Fryery portrait, by Mary Newcomb

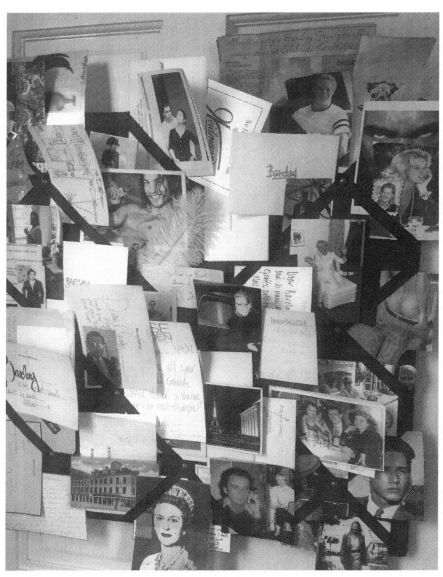

The Memento Board, from the Barclay Fryery Collection

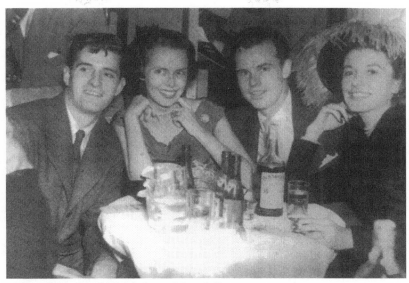

Eileen Ford of Ford Models (second from left)

Cherished, weathered notes from famous editors and the fashion elite frame the bathroom mirror. "Barclay—Your story looks fabulous. Hope you are pleased. I know Mr. POOH will be! So many thanks for the beautiful orchid. Xox," writes Carolyn Sollis, Executive Editor of *House Beautiful*. From Margaret Russell, Editor-in-Chief of *Elle Decor*, in 2001: "Dearest Barclay—Many, many thanks for the terrific star ornament from my favorite star designer!" Senga Mortimer pens, "You spoil me! What a dear you are and so gracious. Thank you sweet Barclay—I love my present and you." Clearly Barclay's gifts extend beyond design to literal gifts, thoughtfully selected and appreciated by their recipients. At a time when it may feel like you can't give as much and mostly need to seek out the kindness of others (from day-to-day care to GoFundMe donations), remembering the chapters of life when you did give—copiously—helps.

There is an invite for "Monsieur Barclay Fryery" to the Chanel show in Paris, reminding him of the front-row seat on a fabulous life he enjoyed for so many years.

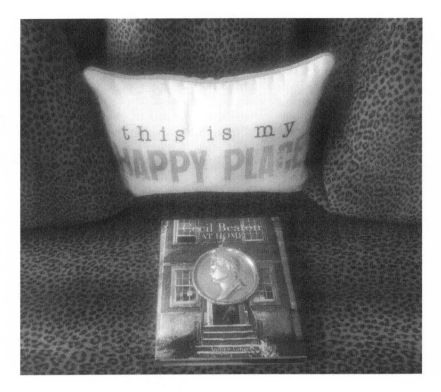

A quilted pillow on the living room couch declares: "This is my HAPPY PLACE."

Part of what makes it that most certainly is the presence of Barclay's calico cat, Princess Royale, who has a crown embroidered on her bed. She purrs through the day, warming herself in the sunrays that fall across Barclay's bedroom and periodically hops down to rub the length of her body across Barclay's calf, blissfully oblivious to his pain and encouraging him to forget it as he tickles behind her ears. Mr. Pooh (the third Mr. Pooh) recently went to a new home with Kate Cherry, the director of the Meridian Museum of Art and one of the three "angels" who care for Barclay. "I couldn't walk him anymore, which is why I gave him another home. It broke my heart because my dog was my baby," says Barclay. But part of his happiness formula is con-

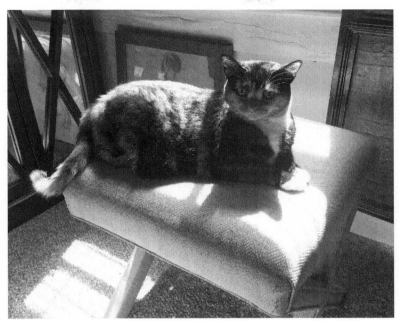

Barclay's cat: Princess Royale

sidering the needs of those around him, including his beloved Mr. Pooh.

LESSON #3: MAKE SOMEONE ELSE FEEL GOOD. There is nothing worse than feeling like a burden. But Barclay's charm and genuine interest in every person he encounters always tip the balance from burden to blessing, even if that person is a nurse changing the dressings on his unsightly feet.

It's easy, if you are suffering, to lash out at those around you. To be grumpy and nasty. It's easy, even if you aren't suffering, to ignore service people, or be rude and demanding. That just isn't— and never was—Barclay's style. I can't count how many times Barclay has told me, "Mama always taught us: Treat the maid the same as the princess." He lives by that rule.

"It's amazing what a little bit of kindness can do. It opens up doors," says Barclay, who has befriended clerks at Walgreens and CVS—invited them over, given them gifts. "They work hard! They are human beings!" exclaims Barclay. He adds, "There are many homeless people here. I don't have a lot of money, but I have enough to treat them to chips and a soda."

Renae comments, "Barclay is kind to everyone. We called him 'sweet grumpy' in the hospital. He knew everyone's name there."

For Barclay, it's just logical. "Being nice to people made the stay easier," he says. "One day Lisa, the head nurse, was having the worst day of her life. I was nice to her and I treated her like a human being, which most people don't do in the hospital. So then she friended me on Facebook and wrote me a lovely note, thanking me for inspiring her to go on."

The "Angels" chapter will elaborate on how being kind through the years has brought so many blessings back to Barclay, especially in this trying time in his life.

LESSON #4: GET UP AND PLAN YOUR DAY. Even though Barclay cannot spring out of bed and go for a run, he has a morning routine that primes him for positive thinking: "I get up, stretch, shower, make my bed, and throw my wash in the laundry. I have to sit down and rest between chores, but I am ready and organized around 7:30 in the morning." Barclay has a loose definition of "showering" now, as the traditional approach is "torture—I'm like the Hunchback of Notre Dame trying to take a shower." French baths are easiest. After all, "the Parisians do it all the time," he notes cheerily. Even this hardship he manages to romanticize. Positive thinking—it's key!

"Choo, Renae, and Kate alternate coming in a couple hours a day. We spend time talking and have dinner or lunch together one on one. We have coffee. I get up and make a latte. It's nice to do something and not just sit here like a vegetable. I have my classical music or opera playing on Pandora 24-7. Pandora saved my sanity. It's supposed to be healing, classical music—Bach and Mozart and Chopin . . . I love Chopin! I'm surrounded by my magazines and books—everything at my fingertips. My cell phone is next to me and people call all day. I keep my house organized so I feel special. I invite people over daily for coffee. I try to have lunch here with someone. I have them choose a book to take from my library. It makes me happy. Gifts arrive, cards arrive, text messages arrive. I try to blog every day."

Though Barclay has faced some criticism for over-sharing on social media during his cancer journey, he firmly believes that being open has helped him. The slew of encouraging comments from his thousands of Facebook friends validates his point. "When I first got sick, everyone stayed away," says Barclay. "Then I put it all out there on Facebook. I'm sharing with the world my journey. That helps me get over the sadness. It's a distraction from all that,

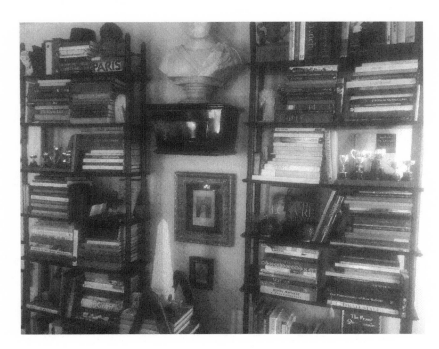

and it dissipates the fear—so people aren't afraid to call me, to visit. People have come forward with other diseases. Cancer survivors have written to me. They've sent books and carpe diems and home remedies from everywhere, from Brazil to Wilton, Connecticut." The openness results in a deluge of advice; Barclay takes it all in, then makes his own decisions.

Eating is difficult but Barclay enjoys lunching, as he always did, and incorporates it into his day. He orders us delicious salads from Harvest Grill. "Make sure it's chopped up really nicely. These New Yorkers don't like big pieces of lettuce," he explains as he orders mine. (I'm actually not averse to a chunky salad, but it's adorable how Barclay attends to every detail to make sure his guests are content.) He orders his with "triple blue cheese" and a baby filet on the side, "cut into little pieces" (he explains that his throat is constricted from cancer—again, he is not afraid to be blunt and in this way he avoids any awkwardness around his illness). "I eat some things, like steak, that I shouldn't," comments Barclay, "because it's fun. I can't turn into a birdseed eater at the end. If I were 30 years younger, absolutely. But I'm 56. I've eaten steak my entire life, and I know it's not good for me, and I'm going to continue eating steak."

Barclay has concluded, after much investigation, that there is no secret weapon to fighting cancer. But a friend has sent a potion, which he is drinking hopefully. "It won't save me," he admits, "but it might prolong my life so I have time to wrap up my life, to finish it."

The way he approaches that is to get up each day with the same plan he has always lived by: "To be the very best I can be."

LESSON #5: KEEP YOUR SENSE OF HUMOR. Sure, cancer is no laughing matter, but that doesn't mean laughing won't help you through it. Among the portraits and paintings on Barclay's living room wall, I stumble upon this gem of a sign: "Your crazy

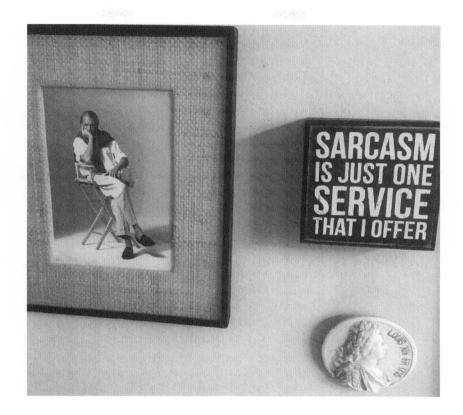

is showing. You might want to tuck that back in." I can picture Barclay in stylist mode, chasing after nutty family members and friends, tucking in their crazy . . . and their catty . . . and snooty . . . and nasty . . . and grumpy. It would actually be quite useful to have stylists not only for our outfits and our hair but also for our personalities!

Another sign reads: "Sarcasm is just one service that I offer." In addition, some of you may be lucky enough to know that Barclay continues to offer singing voice mail services. When he wakes up feeling crappy, Barclay doesn't pick up the phone and bitch. He actually calls up friends and treats them to a little tune—often morning coffee-themed—sung in the melodious voice he inherited from his mom, who briefly was a professional singer (until his

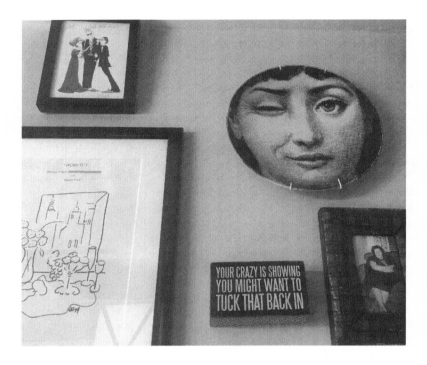

father, Lee Fryery, forbade her from performing, but that's a story for another chapter).

"They are all original compositions," notes Barclay, a baritone trained in musical theatre (also an activity forbidden by his father). "I don't like to do anything humdrum." Renae played me one from her phone, which ends in an operatic flourish:

> *If you're happy and you know it, sip some coffee,*
> *sip, sip,*
> *If you're happy and you know it, sip some coffee,*
> *sip, sip,*
> *If you're happy and you know it, then your cup will*
> *really show it.*
> *Coffeeeeeeeeeeee, sipppppppyyy, sipppppppyyy!*

These ditties definitely do not sound like the work of a dying man. They are not. They are the work of a living man. One who is sucking every bit of liveliness out of every minute.

I now have several personalized Barclay tunes saved on my phone for posterity, never to be deleted. For me, he added tea, my breakfast drink of choice, to a lovely 34-second ballad. Thoughtful, creative, funny—take that, cancer!

By the way, morning caffeine is not the only topic in Barclay's songbook. He's also big on poop songs. Yep, preschoolers would love this, but so does another demographic. "The diarrhea and constipation that comes with cancer and radiation is something no one talks about. The diarrhea for three months, the constipation for six months—it's *horrible*," states Barclay. "So you gotta have fun with it. What else can you do?"

Barclay launches in, "How is your poop this morning? Is yours tall, dark, and handsome?" Then he adds, "No, it was the log ride at Six Flags! Now when I'm talking to my closest friends, I'll say, 'I was on the log ride today. It was something else!' You know South Park had a little poop character that sang show tunes. I loved him." Insert poop emoji here ☺.

If only all the shit we will delve into in coming chapters were as silly as that!

CHAPTER 2

Demons

——◦—◦——◦—◦—

Abused, Bullied, Suicidal—A Gay Boy
Builds a Fortress for Life

WHEN I DROVE THE HOUR FROM THE airport in Jackson to Barclay's hometown of Meridian—a straight-shot across Interstate 20—my mind occasionally was drawn away from dear Barclay and his disease to pondering the complex and sometimes horrific history of the South. Scenes from *The Help* scrolled through my brain. I'm not often in the South, particularly the Deep South, so the past seems all the more palpable. It hangs in the air with the humidity. I have to push through it to be in the present more than in other places.

But this story I'd tell with Barclay would not be a dark *Prince of Tides*-type affair. It would be more like a *Vanity Fair* affair, up until cancer came and spoiled the party. At least so I thought.

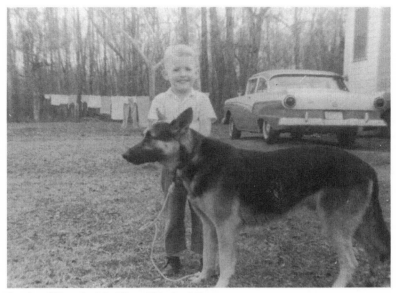

Barclay ("Timothy Mark") and his dog Mister

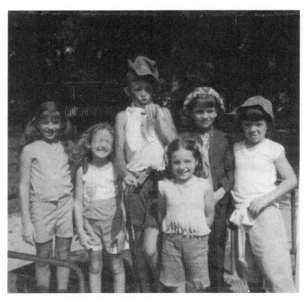

Barclay (middle) at his Hobo Birthday Party

Timothy Mark Fryery was born on August 5, 1960. He was an adorable child, a towhead with a sweet grin. As a toddler, he sat on Santa's knee at Sears and Roebuck and asked for a baby sister. Lisa Fryery arrived just before the following Christmas. "I cherished her," says Barclay. "She was my baby doll. Because she had red hair and freckles, the bully in the neighborhood said she was ugly and called her a skunk. I said, 'Oh no, she's my ladybug!'" The nickname stuck; Lisa is still "Bug" to Barclay, and she calls him "Brother Love."

Lisa stops by during my visit and brings our lunch. "Oh here's my bug!" exclaims Barclay. "She's my bug, isn't she cute?"

"You feel good 'cause you had company coming, huh?" says Lisa, giving him a hug. She's as gracious as her brother, and as beautiful as he is handsome.

Barclay tells his sister how we met, how we connected as editor and writer, then lost touch. "Facebook brought everyone together. It's amazing," says Barclay. He tells her about our book, and where the name came from. "When I saw Jill last spring for lunch in Greenwich, she said, 'Cancer looks good on you.'" With a wry grin, Barclay adds, "I responded, 'Well, looks were never my problem.'" Bug claps her hands together and laughs.

Like Barclay, Lisa is stylish. She apologizes for her flip-flops (fine with me) and frizzy hair (not compared to mine) from working in the plant. Barclay explains that she runs a drycleaner. "I have some sandals I'm going to change into," she says. Her outfit incorporates a belt he gave her, a gold ring with a big red pendant from Barclay, and a ring from her dad. "My tough-guy rings," she says.

"I gave her all of my belts because my waist ballooned up," Barclay explains.

These gifts, from a wardrobe that is being whittled down deliberately due to an impending lack of need on this Earth, are as far as Lisa can go in accepting what's ahead.

"I love you. Get back to work," says Barclay, when it's time for her to go. "I love you with all my heart." With some recent burglaries in the neighborhood in mind, he calls after her, "I'm being Lee Fryery now: be very aware of your surroundings." It's clear the pair adore each other.

"I reserve time with her for fun things, for laughter," explains Barclay. "She has gone through a tough 10 years of going through a divorce, helping with my father and my mother, raising teenage boys. I don't want to burden her more. She put up an emotional wall at first because she didn't want to see me go. I'm her only sibling. The Fryerys are all very stoic on the outside but inside we are marshmallows. She's not ready to say good-bye."

When I learn more of their childhood story, I understand why. Denial is a family coping mechanism, and so this is how Bug deals with Barclay's disease.

> *"The Fryerys are all very stoic on the outside but inside we are marshmallows."*

DISEASE IS NOT NEW TO THE FAMILY. Their dear mother, Frances Fryery, sadly developed Alzheimer's 15 years ago, at the age of 64. "When I started losing her, I lost my best friend in the whole world. She was my rock," says Barclay. "All she can think of now is her 'baby boy.' She doesn't remember many other people. She wants to make me minute steak, garlic mashed potatoes, snap green beans, and give me lunch. That's all she can think about. Bug walked in on her pleading with God not to take her baby boy. She and I are very close. I shared everything with her. I spoiled her. She can't ever know I'm sick. She knows I have something but can't

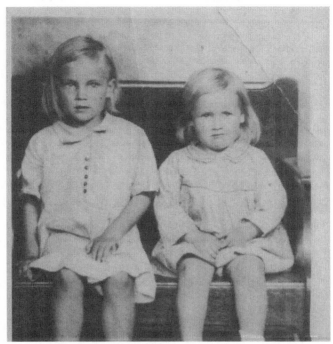

Barclay's mother, Frances (right), with her sister Grace, circa 1941

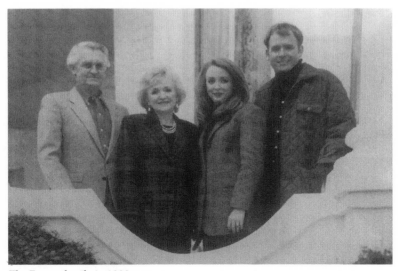

The Fryery family in 1998

know that it's fatal. I've told her that I've broken my leg and that's why I'm not visiting."

Born Emma Frances Anthony, Frances's stage name was Jeanie Francis, back when she was singing in a band and on the radio in Jackson. "She's a tiny, petite thing," says Barclay. "I used to call her Jeanie Vanity Fryery when she was acting vain." One of Barclay's fondest memories is "drinking Diet Coke and eating Funyuns when we watched the soap operas with Mama. That was our indulgence."

I ask to see a picture of his parents. "Yes, take a look in the kitchen," he says. "There are all kinds of pictures around of my mother, my sister, and me. Not too many of my daddy." I find one of the family, taken almost 20 years ago. They are a handsome, perfectly styled family.

"Mother taught us: If you have one white shirt, a pair of pants, a bar of soap, your nails clean, and your hair combed, you will never be a hot mess," explains Barclay. Mama's life lessons had a profound influence on his code of conduct. A closet packed with dozens of crisp white shirts, still in their dry-cleaning plastic, suggests Barclay took this particular lesson a tad far, but he lives by a "what if?" mentality—also engrained by Mama. So *what if* he happened to spill ketchup on 155 of the 156 shirts in the closet? He'd still safely avoid hot mess status.

> *"Mother taught us: If you have one white shirt, a pair of pants, a bar of soap, your nails clean, and your hair combed, you will never be a hot mess."*

"We were always taught to have things picked up in the house, because what if guests come? I raked the shag carpet. We set the table. Our room was clean and our toys put away," continues Bar-

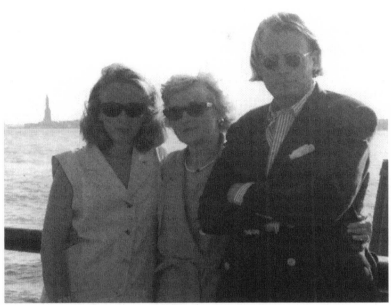

Barclay with his mother, Frances, and sister, Lisa ("Bug")

clay. "We were taught to be neat and tidy in public." This helped Barclay in his career. Perhaps it also helped his mother cover up the parts of their lives that were not so neat and tidy in private.

Lee Fryery, Barclay's father, was a hardworking man. He was a fireman, truck driver, and jack-of-all-trades. He made sure he provided for his family. He built the house in which Barclay grew up, a simple Sears and Roebuck-designed ranch. "Everyone thinks if you come from the South, you grew up in a grand antebellum mansion with columns," says Barclay. "My childhood home was a beige and white, three-bedroom/two-bath, with air conditioning units in the windows. It was anything but what I evolved to. It was lovely and charming in our eyes, though. There were lots of poor people in Meridian who lived beyond the railroad tracks, where sewage flooded every time it rained. To Bug and me, our house was a mansion. And it was always neat and organized and decorated."

Before Barclay was born, Lee Fryery yearned for a son. "He told my mom, 'Everyone's got a little boy. I want one,'" explains Barclay. "But he did not get the kind of boy he wanted."

Barclay liked Boy Scouts, rock and coin collecting, playing in the woods—boyish activities. But he also liked theater and decorated his room a certain way. "I was not a sissy boy, but to him I was, and that made him angry," says Barclay. "Out hunting, I would skim rocks and scare the deer away. It just wasn't my thing. On fishing trips, I'd talk and scare the fish away."

Lee Fryery took a Southern approach to the problem: he would beat it out of his son. "He dressed me up in a fireman's uniform and paraded me around the front yard," says Barclay, straining to think of a happy memory with his dad, "but the very next week, he backhanded me for squinting in the sun when taking a photo."

Barclay is hesitant about revealing abuse he has not shared with anyone until this final chapter in his life. He does not want to disgrace his family. But when we talk about other young gay people, faced with their parents' and society's intolerance, Barclay realizes that telling his story—showing where he came from and what he became—will help others. Helping trumps honor. It is not from a vindictive or bitter place that the stories begin tumbling out.

"He beat the hell out of me every chance he could, until I left home," he says. "And many gay

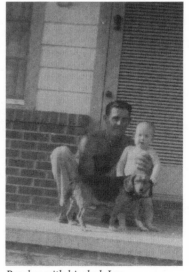

Barclay with his dad, Lee

people go through that, and I didn't even know I was gay. I didn't even know what the word meant, but he thought I was gay. Or I'm not sure he knew exactly what it was, but there was something that made me different: the way I styled my room, the way I wore my clothes. I wanted to be in theater and model. He beat me like a dog, in front of people. I remember him hitting me on my Aunt Evelyn's property, until—and this sounds crazy, like *The Beverly Hillbillies*—she yelled, 'If you hit that young boy one more time, I'll kill you!'

"My father raised hunting dogs. When he could not catch me to beat me, he would, for no reason, beat them unmercifully. The entire neighborhood would hear in disbelief. He had them caged, then chained. Many of them would jump over the fencing to try to escape, thus hanging themselves in the process." Barclay understood the animals' desperate impulse.

"You have dos and don'ts in life. Suicide is a don't. . . . You have let them win if you choose that option. All your work and dreams are done then."

"As a kid, I was going to kill myself many times. I could not do that to my mother. So I did not," says Barclay, whose resolve as a boy has carried over into another time when ending the suffering inevitably comes to mind. "You have dos and don'ts in life," states Barclay. "Suicide is a don't. It's not an option. It should be considered with all you are going through if you are in my position, but you have let them win if you choose that option. All your work and dreams are done then. That's not my last chapter.

"If you are bullied and ostracized as I was, you have to get thick skin and plow right through. Never let your eyes off theirs. The Leo is the king of the jungle; I'm not going to wallow, absolutely not. It takes guts to remove that option from the table once and for all. Unfortunately, it's the path that many people take. I want to wrap my arms around all of them." From his Facebook posts to this book to a lifetime of random acts of kindness, Barclay metaphorically does wrap his arms around all of them—every outsider, gay person, abused kid, cancer sufferer, and hospice patient.

"If you are bullied and ostracized as I was, you have to get thick skin and plow right through. Never let your eyes off theirs."

WHEN BARCLAY TALKS ABOUT BULLYING, he is not only referring to his dad. High school was no joy ride for an effeminate boy from a small Sears and Roebuck ranch who yearned to hang out with the rich kids. "When we were little, our neighborhood seemed upper middle class to us. As puberty set in, we started integrating into bigger schools. We saw Mercedes and Jaguars for the first time and fancy houses in a neighborhood we'd never visited before. Rich and poor children attended school together but kept very much in their station.

"I of course gravitated toward the rich children, because they were more interesting in my mind's eye. They were anything but welcoming. Then I realized I was not 'as good as they were.' So I began to get dropped off two blocks earlier and walk home. It was the first time I felt socio-economic shame. Kids began to drive by on the weekends, blowing their horns, letting me know they knew where I lived. It was very similar to *Pretty in Pink*. I sewed buttons on my shirts to make them button-downs to fit in; she made her own clothes. When I watched that movie I thought, *Wow, there are so many parallels to my youth.* It is a fabulous movie about the social dynamics of a town."

At a young age, Barclay discovered a cultural and psychological escape. "At school and at the Meridian Little Theatre, I found an outlet in theater because it mixed children together of all backgrounds. When I got a part over a rich kid, I would chuckle inside. John Hall, my biggest nemesis, got the one-line part of Tigger in *Winnie the Pooh*. I got the big role of the wise Owl. Society wasn't choosing me; the director was. In theater, I could be anything I wanted to be and no one was going to hold me back. I was in every play and musical there was from age 7. I got standing ovations. I was a good actor. I danced and sang—I sang like a lark. I was judged for my merit, not what my father did for a living." Barclay also was part of singing groups, the Lamplighters in high school and Variations in junior college. "We sang at the National Junior Miss Pageant in Mobile, which was a big deal," notes Barclay.

"In theater, I could be anything I wanted to be and no one was going to hold me back."

However, Barclay's father did not approve of his son being a thespian, and singing and dancing were not considered appropriate. Disapproval sometimes came in the form of bruises and welts in the Fryery home. "I had to sneak away to try out for plays. My parents wouldn't find out until the pictures hit the newspapers. The director was gay (secretly, of course, back then, but people knew). So they thought everyone was gay. My father was controlling. My mother used to be a singer and she modeled. He was jealous of her and went to Jackson and took her off the radio. She cut one album and then he made her stop. I love my mother very much. She was a bystander. My father was the culprit. My sister— I protected. I took all the lickings for her. Daddy worshipped her.

"Our house was filled only with religion, and we were told we could do nothing else. We went to an Evangelical church. They weren't handling rattlesnakes for God's sake, and there were families there that were fine, but my parents took an all-religious—not a Christian—take on things. So everything was a sin. I would go to school dances and be followed. I would go to parties and they would call the house 60 times and embarrass me, so I'd never see those friends again." His mother modeled charitable behavior, though, and that is the pattern gentle Barclay followed, not one of abuse.

"My father had a very poor sister who was raped by an older man when she was 12," recounts Barclay. "Of course she was accused of seducing him, and she lost her mind. She married a simple man. We weren't allowed to mix with them, which is the typical southern approach if a side of the family is really poor. My mother would pack up the Delta 88 white Oldsmobile and take clothes and food secretly to them, because my father was embarrassed. She tried to minister to them through kindness; I learned that from her. She and Lisa Bug and I would go there all the time—not to have dinner

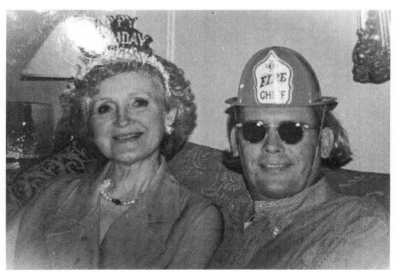

Barclay with his beautiful mom

or socialize, because they didn't understand us either, but just to take them things they needed. My mother is a wonderful person."

Barclay and Lisa have bequeathed their mother's bedroom furniture to the daughter of that aunt. The house itself they need to cover the cost of the home for Alzheimer's patients, where their mother is cared for now. "It's quite lovely," says Barclay. "It has a real dining room, library, and drawing room. She has no concept of where she is. She thinks her husband is still at home and she has to go take care of him."

He is not at home and was plagued by dementia in his twilight years as well. We will get to the details of who actually took care of him later. For now, consider that perhaps one disease is relief from another. Barclay's brain, with cancer, remains as sharp as it was when he plotted his escape from his childhood hell.

Barclay now sits on the Board of Directors of the Meridian Little Theatre. He also sits in a fortress he began building way back then. It is a place from which you can wake up, stare cancer in the face, and then phone a friend and sing them a morning coffee song.

Barclay's final performance while still living at home is seared in his mind due to the incident that preceded it. "I was 18 and attending junior college at the time, because my parents didn't think I was responsible enough to go away to school yet," explains Barclay. "I was performing in *Side by Side* by Sondheim. My dad hit me in the head with a galvanized metal garbage can lid for an hour before a show because he didn't want me performing. It may as well have been a hammer. Our minister's wife, Dot Frasier, realized what had happened. She held my hand through makeup. I had to go on and sing 'Marry Me a Little,' a very difficult song to sing, as Sondheim songs always are. I didn't miss a beat.

"A gun was put to my head the last day before I left. I didn't come home for years, but I sent presents, because you want to try to buy love."

Barclay now sits on the Board of Directors of the Meridian Little Theatre. He also sits in a fortress he began building way back then. It is a place from which you can wake up, stare cancer in the face, and then phone a friend and sing them a morning coffee song.

"When you've been through all I've been through as a child and put up walls to protect yourself and then you climb over the walls," says Barclay, "you can't give up."

CHAPTER 3

Reinvention

What You Gotta Do Is Dream BIG!

BARCLAY TRAVELED THE WORLD as a boy, but only in his mind. He would go to the mall and pore over all kinds of magazines. "Through magazines I traveled to all regions," says Barclay. "I educated myself that way. Watching movies—inclusive ones—and documentaries is a great way to learn and broaden your viewpoint."

The first time Barclay really got away from the confines of a small-town mentality and out from under the thumb of his disapproving father was when he headed to college at the University of Mississippi. "I had a wonderful time at Ole Miss," says Barclay, talking now as if a shadow has lifted as he moves into this next chapter of his life. "I was president of my pledge class at Phi Kappa Tau."

Barclay's best friend from college, Daniel Lavon Herrington ("DL" to Barclay), happens to call while I'm interviewing him. Barks passes the phone my way and Daniel launches into stories from the good *ole* days: "I first saw Barclay in the student union. He was the most starched person on a campus of starched people. Every pleat was crisp. Later that week, there was a knock at my door. And he's standing there, perfectly over-starched. He started to say, 'I'm running for . . .' and I slammed the door. Then we got to be friends. We were like the Bobbsey twins. We were up for everything that was going on."

"He was the most starched person on a campus of starched people. Every pleat was crisp."

Barclay was studying English literature and French, but he was cultivating his design skills too. "His dorm room was just immaculate," says Daniel, "and he had designed it with a sofa, chairs, and pillows. I think it was the only designer dorm room on campus!"

A year into their friendship, Daniel transferred to Millsaps College in Jackson. "Barclay started to visit me on weekends," continues Daniel. "At that time, he was very Republican. I was very outrageous. I was a club kid before the concept of club kids even came to Mississippi. It was a very unlikely relationship.

"One night we were getting ready to head out to the bars in Memphis. I'd been given some Yves St. Laurent bronzer for Christmas (this was back before anyone knew about bronzer). It was springtime and Barclay decided we should go in tennis whites with Louis Vuitton bags. I put on the bronzer. Barclay insisted, 'I want some, I want some.' He comes back 45 minutes later and the new tube is empty. You see how white he is! Later on the dance floor, sweat was running off him and white lines were forming down his face and bronzer was splattering all over everyone on the dance floor! His white shirt looked like it had blood all over it." Daniel is chuckling as he tells the story. "I just stood off to the side and laughed. I didn't tell him."

Barclay, for once in his life, may have looked a hot mess, but he was a happy mess. He didn't hold the incident against his devilish pal. "We have stayed in touch all through the years," says Daniel.

Barclay gushes, "Daniel taught me everything. He was my Dr. Frankenstein. He created me. Back then, he resembled Gary Numan, the punk rocker. We were an odd match. Now he's preppy like me. He's a wonderful man. Daniel taught me how to be a gentleman and be gay. We talk every day. His mother was my Big Mama (from *Cat on a Hot Tin Roof*). She took me under her wing and was like a second mom to me."

"I didn't want to be held back by what people said I was, so I changed my name. Why can't you choose a name?

From the age of 8, young "Timothy Mark" had been scribbling down different names, contemplating a new identity. "Being gay was taboo in Meridian. It still is. I didn't want to be held back by what people said I was," explains Barclay, "so I changed my name, like Cary Grant did. He was Archibald Leach; who wants that name? Why can't you choose a name? A king chooses a name; before he is crowned, he chooses which name he wants to go by. I didn't want to be stuck with a name that had a stigma to it. I was held back because I came from a middle-class neighborhood. I was held back because my dad was a fire chief. I was held back because of the church I went to. Gosh darn it, I was going to go out and discover the world and let the world discover a fresh spirit. And they weren't going to hold me back. I figured, if the world would embrace me, then my hometown would."

In Meridian, Barclay was labeled as "other," but the label he coveted was "special." He would pick a name that was unique and sounded special—and, whether he knew it or not then, a name that would be catchy should the implausible happen: that a bullied boy from Mississippi might one day become a brand. In 1982, after he graduated from Ole Miss, Timothy Mark Fryery became *Barclay Fryery*. He legally changed his name in 1991 (incidentally the year I graduated from college and underwent my own reinvention, but that is a whole other book).

I have another friend who had a rough childhood and chose to change her name as well. Though that was partly to evade her abuser, it also created a blank slate, a new beginning. Empowered with his new identity, Barclay headed east and left Timothy Mark behind. For the most part, he wouldn't need Timothy again, though there was one more burden Timothy would have to carry in the future.

"What you gotta do is dream big, as big as you want, and then grow into it," says Barclay. "It's like decorating: pull out all the stops and then edit down to what you can handle. Then move a little bit, take baby steps." Someone might have given Ronald Reagan the same advice in his youth, and by 1982, when Barclay moved to DC, the actor-turned-politician was in the White House. Talk about reinvention. (Granted, by 2016, Reagan would no longer seem like such an unconventional candidate!)

"What you gotta do is dream big, as big as you want, and then grow into it. It's like decorating: pull out all the stops and then edit down to what you can handle. Then move a little bit, take baby steps."

Barclay decided to go to Washington because "that's where I thought all the power was," he says. "I was a Young Republican. I'd worked on the Reagan Youth Campaign. At Central Methodist, I'd met Meg Speed, who was the daughter of the richest man in Meridian. Because I was responsible and she was irresponsible, they would send me in a Jag and have me take her to debutante parties and treated me as one of them. He wrote my first recommendation letter. It was glowing. I had done good things," says Barclay. "Due to that letter, I worked for the Reagan Youth Campaign and for College Republicans. I worked in the House of Representatives as an intern for Sunny Montgomery, who was gay as well (he wasn't out).

"When I went back to DC in '82, I worked at RNC, Republican National Committee. I got my feet wet in politics. But the more I learned about politics, the more I didn't want to be in politics. So I went back to my fashion roots."

Barclay had worked at a men's store in Meridian. "I was the buyer, model, window dresser—I did everything, including selling," he says. "It was an ultra-preppy store. I was so good that the owner offered to back my own store when I graduated from Ole Miss. But I wanted to go see more in the world." Barclay landed a gig in DC organizing and styling a photo shoot. The results, of course, were fabulous.

Socially, Barclay discovered the international melting pot in the capitol and began frequenting Café Med, where he danced up to his waist in packing bubbles, and Desiree—"a really chic club at the Four Seasons. I went with the Egyptian Prince Osman Ibrahami and his entourage. I kind of just fit in. If you smile and look pulled together, they accept you and bring you into their pack. I had done the Waspy Georgetown thing, but my big swoop into the design world was through this international circle. Washington was a lot of fun in the late '70s and early '80s. I saw all kinds of fashion and met all types of people."

At 23, Barclay went to lunch with someone he considered to be his best friend at the time, Bradley Whitehurst. "I told him, 'I want to be a designer,'" says Barclay, "and he laughed at me! He said, 'You are not being realistic.'"

Barclay was taken aback. But not one to have his dreams shot down, he became even more determined to seek out the top designers in DC. "I met one of them, Anthony Brown, just by coincidence at a party in Key West," says Barclay. "We became friends and he invited me to his parties, where I met all the other fabulous designers. I started contemplating a move to New York."

Let's just take a moment to review here. A few years before this, Timothy Fryery was being tormented by snobby peers and clobbered over the head with a garbage can lid by his dad—basically being sent the message that he and his passions were trash. Now, the new Barclay Fryery is attending fabulous parties in Key West, hobnobbing with royalty, pursuing a field his father would never consider manly enough, and having a marvelous time. This name-change thing is really powerful! Cue the music from *Rocky* when Sly is running up the steps to the Philadelphia Museum of Art (I had to Google where exactly those steps were . . . an art museum—perfect!). Our boy Barclay is breaking out. He's making it!

NOT SO FAST. IT'S KIND OF LIKE with cancer. You wake up one day and feel like you can conquer the world; the next day feels like it might be your last . . . There was another disease simmering around this time, getting ready to boil over and spoil the party and lay waste to the wide-eyed hopes and dreams of boys like Barclay.

"Once the AIDS crisis hit, I was afraid to go to New York," recounts Barclay. "I was afraid I would catch it. Like I did as a child, I would read about New York. I looked at *W, M, Vogue*. I liked coke a bit too much with my international crowd, because that's what was involved with them. And I almost killed myself on that. I checked myself into rehab back in Meridian at the East Mississippi State Hospital—an insane asylum. I chose that because I wanted to be shocked and not go to a glamorous place that my friends could have paid for, where I'd just learn from the rich kids what new drugs to try. I wanted to go to a place that would scare the heck out of me, so I'd never do it again. So I checked in, with drug addicts and convicts. I was the only one like me. We even had a transvestite nurse. It was *One Flew Over the Cuckoo's Nest* times ten."

Barclay never touched a drug again (at least not until the morphine that is required to cope with the pain of terminal cancer). "You don't ever have to tell me more than once, ever, on anything," he says.

CRAVING CULTURE, NOT COKE, Barclay headed to New Orleans next. He got a job as the food and catering director for the Columns Hotel in the Garden District. "I wrote all their menus," says Barclay. "Then I came across an ad in the paper for Barbizon, which I knew was the worst!" (Ah, we are both caught. I fell for a TV ad at age 11!) Barclay had no shortcomings in the looks department, but he was overloaded in the height department. Men as tall as he is are a fit challenge, so he could only dabble in modeling. He mastered posing. Barclay would look dapper and dashing in every photo ever taken of him, even those in which cancer had him in a choke hold.

Barclay began to meet the movers and shakers of New Orleans. "The Barbizon director introduced me to Harris Cohen. He was a big queen, very persnickety, and very rich. He hired me to work at a store, J. Hermann and Sons, to watch his investment there. He gave me an apartment that was an old slave quarter, 333 Royal, which I

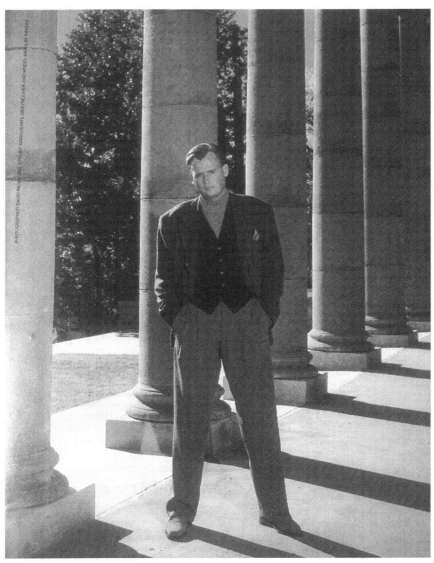

Barclay modeling in New Orleans in 1989

could restore and do whatever to at no charge. He took me to the New Orleans Athletic Club and got me a membership. He took me to supper clubs, with his wife, a princess from Rome. Again, I did nothing but look cute and be a sweet guy. I think because I was treated so badly, I made that my mantra: to be as sweet as I could be and see what happens. It opened doors. It forged friendships, whether with the janitor or royalty. I went to my first black-tie balls. I learned about white tie and tails and everything that went along with that. Of course, New Orleans was a melting pot too: people from New York, people from Europe. I made all kinds of friends.

> *"I made that my mantra: to be as sweet as I could be and see what happens."*

"Then my best friend from my Washington days, Michael Ronkese, sent me a horrific letter telling me he was dying of AIDs. He had a few months to live. I went to take care of him. He had been shunned by friends and his lover had left and moved to New York." Barclay has trouble revisiting these painful memories but continues, "I spent his last week with him in his DC apartment. This was 1990. His body was very white and puffy from the horrible meds then. I was terrified myself, but endured because he was such a positive force in my life and my own coming of age as a young gay man. I loved him like a brother."

Michael, who had been a priest, had, in a way, saved Barclay. He'd helped eradicate yet another horrifying layer of suffering from Barclay's life (which we will explore in the "Angels" chapter).

Barclay buried his friend. The disease was getting closer.

BARCLAY FELT THE NEED AGAIN to start over. He went back to New Orleans, packed up his things, and headed to a town that epitomized the chic life he dreamed of back when the rich kids were honking and harassing him in his middle-class Meridian 'hood.

He had a friend, Bill Romanello, whose parents had a home in Greenwich, Connecticut. He camped out on a spare sofa. "Bill got me a job at Ralph Lauren," says Barclay. "I then did the windows at an Argentine Polo shop called La Martina. I did all the windows at Greenwich Orchids, and the antiques. I ran both stores and styled both." Barclay was not only living in Greenwich, he was literally creating the ideal image of the aspirational life for his fellow residents.

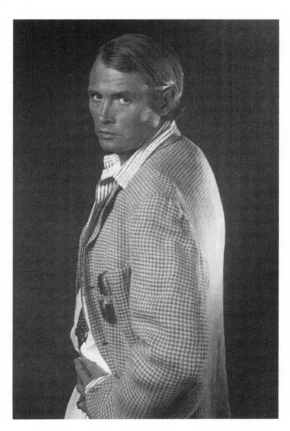

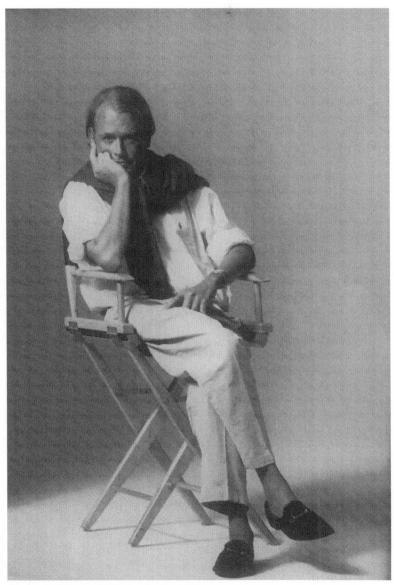

Barclay in Soho in 1996, shot by David Cluett

But when all employees had to do a blood test for Greenwich Orchid's group insurance plan, there was a problem. The health insurance company sent the results through the store's fax machine. "I was out on a delivery, so I came back to Greenwich Orchids and everyone knew before I knew: I was HIV positive." Barclay was fired on the spot.

"I went home and laid on the floor. I lost my apartment. I lost my boyfriend. People were so afraid."

"I went home and laid on the floor. I lost my apartment. I lost my boyfriend. People were so afraid," says Barclay. "I called Christ Church in Greenwich. There was a gay priest there, and he helped me get off the ground. I got into a new apartment on Greenwich Avenue and started over, with an attitude that nothing was going to keep me down."

CHAPTER 4

The Brand

◦—◦—◦—◦—◦

Building a Design Empire

"Good Morning World: Bring It On!"

This is a recent post, from April 18, 2017, on Barclay's Facebook page. Clearly, he is determined to go out with a roar, not a whimper.

Had Facebook been around, Barclay very well may have posted the same challenge to the world back in 1991. He had a new stigmatizing label: *HIV positive*. Friends and colleagues ostracized him. He knew he might die. But he found a way to compartmentalize that reality so that he did not give up on life. Barclay had all the more reason to get busy and make his mark.

> *Friends and colleagues ostracized him. He knew he might die. But he found a way to compartmentalize that reality so that he did not give up on life.*

"When I became HIV positive, almost 30 years ago, I did not admit it to myself," says Barclay. "Timothy Mark had HIV and could get AIDS and Barclay Fryery did not. That kept me sane. That's how I divided up the sickness." Thankfully, it was 1991 and medicine had come a long way since the early years of the AIDS crisis. While a potent cocktail of medication kept Barclay alive for decades, he wonders if the treatment—perhaps rushed onto the market without thorough trials—caused his cancer. He wonders; he does not wallow.

Likewise, in the 1990s, Barclay did anything but wallow. He was hired to help at a garden show. "I sold $25,000 worth of jardinière urns in one day, and that started my career," he says. "A few years later Albert Hadley was the judge of the Southport Garden Festival, and I did Lovey and Thurston Howell's hut from *Gilligan's Island,* with the music and everything. He told me, 'Nice job, kiddo,'" recounts Barclay. Hadley, a design icon, became a mentor and they developed a friendship. "I asked him, 'Albert, how do I get published?' I had no idea.

"The next day he invited me to a dinner party and sat me next to *Elle Decor* editor Marian McEvoy. She actually liked me and I liked her. I let it sit for a while and simmer. I was on the Antiquarius committee in Greenwich, and I chose her to lecture," explains Barclay. "After the lecture—which was quite wonderful—I asked her, 'Do you have five minutes to come see my apartment?' We entered the building and my partner's Boxer had shit all over his apartment! So I couldn't show her his work. I showed her my apartment and the office, and she told me, 'Let's do it! You'll hear from Margaret Russell.' Margaret was the assistant editor at that time."

Barclay and his chic one-bedroom Greenwich Avenue apartment were published in *Elle Decor*'s small features section in 1998. Even Mr. Pooh (Mr. Pooh II) made the spread, along with his debonair master. It was a highpoint of Barclay's budding design

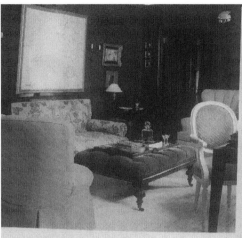

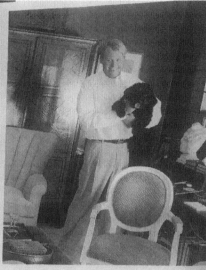

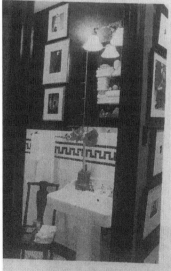

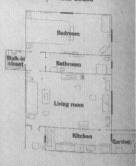

Barclay Fryery is a landlord's dream tenant. Not only did he design, oversee, and finance major improvements on his 900-square-foot rental apartment in Greenwich, Connecticut, he even redecorated the building's shared space, placing mounted antlers from his father's hunting-trophy collection over his neighbors' doorways, for instance, and springing for brass doorplates. "I basically took over," says Fryery. In return, his landlord offered him extra storage space under the stairs.

Colors and textures—two components that the interior designer believes are paramount to living with style in small quarters—dominate the flat. The walls are painted red, chocolate-brown, black, and white; Edwardian-style furnishings, some upholstered in Manuel Canovas yellows and reds, mix with Federal pieces; and the bedroom is covered from floor to ceiling in black-and-white Waverly ticking.

There was no kitchen, so Fryery installed a smart little kitchenette with mirrored walls and a few appliances: a microwave, a compact Sub-Zero refrigerator, a fax machine, and a word processor. (He never cooks and instead uses the space as a home office.) also made an utterly nondescript ba room glamorous, painting the wa black and decorating with framed ph tographs and old-world details, like cut-glass doorknob and a Greek-k patterned tile border. "I restored eve thing in the apartment," says Fryery, even had the radiators taken out a lacquered white. There wasn't a wh lot of aesthetics here, so I had to ma something wonderful out of nothing— bit of Thomas Jefferson living in 20th century." **Julia Szabo**

Barclay's Greenwich apartment in Elle Decor

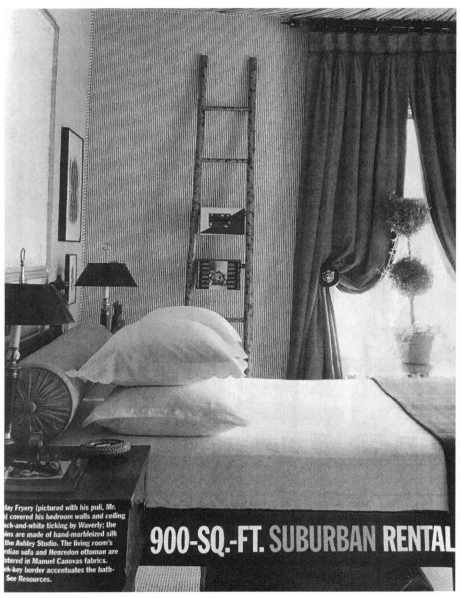

day Fryery (pictured with his puli, Mr.
) covered his bedroom walls and ceiling
ack-and-white ticking by Waverly; the
ins are made of hand-marbleized silk
the Ashley Studio. The living room's
rdian sofa and Henredon ottoman are
stered in Manuel Canovas fabrics.
ek-key border accentuates the bath-
See Resources.

900-SQ.-FT. SUBURBAN RENTAL

Barclay's bedroom in Elle Decor

career. "Once you are published by a great magazine, others want to see what you are doing, and people want to hire you," notes Barclay. Not surprisingly, many career high points followed:

BEING PUBLISHED IN *HOUSE BEAUTIFUL* IN 2002

This feature, entitled "Darkness Visible," included Barclay's exquisite fire escape garden and 300 (!) red roses in a square vase on his coffee table, with a grinning Mr. Pooh posed beside it. "From his unprepossessing perch in suburban Greenwich, Connecticut, decorator Barclay Fryery ups the drama quotient with basic black," reads the subhead. The details: "Weatherproof Sunbrella fabric in bright Matisse colors covers tuffets on the tiny terrace, framed by 19th-century wrought-iron gates. The living room's dark walls and light floors, painted with Ralph Lauren's Black Panther and Dover Cliffs, provide a sophisticated backdrop for a 19th-century corner chair and the Anglo-Indian ottoman from Henredon. Ralph Lauren's Regimental Blue paint sparks the foyer walls." I want to move right in; how about you?

BEING ON *HOUSE WARS* IN 2003

In this show, each star interior decorator was assigned to a family and given a $10,000 budget per room to overhaul a house—which the victorious family got to keep. Barclay was assigned to the Dahm family. They had been on several reality shows, as well as *Family Feud*, and the bombshell Dahm triplets appeared in *Playboy* in 1998 (one of them would go on to marry the son of Dr. Phil). The show was shot in Phoenix in July, so Barclay devised a strategy: "I went to Africa in the middle of July to condition my body to that horrible heat and to see the vibrant colors and red clay of Marrakech. I chose desert colors—a Moroccan color scheme—not American colors. We won! I am still friends with the Dahm triplets. They are really quite wonderful girls."

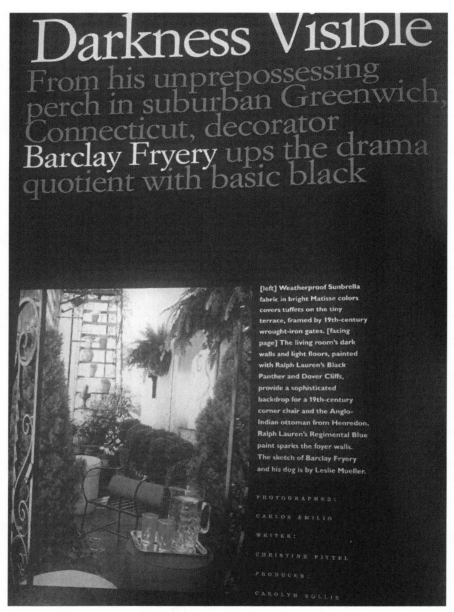

Darkness Visible

From his unprepossessing perch in suburban Greenwich, Connecticut, decorator Barclay Fryery ups the drama quotient with basic black

[left] Weatherproof Sunbrella fabric in bright Matisse colors covers tuffets on the tiny terrace, framed by 19th-century wrought-iron gates. [facing page] The living room's dark walls and light floors, painted with Ralph Lauren's Black Panther and Dover Cliffs, provide a sophisticated backdrop for a 19th-century corner chair and the Anglo-Indian ottoman from Henredon. Ralph Lauren's Regimental Blue paint sparks the foyer walls. The sketch of Barclay Fryery and his dog is by Leslie Mueller.

PHOTOGRAPHER:

CARLOS EMILIO

WRITER:

CHRISTINE PITTEL

PRODUCER:

CAROLYN SOLLIS

Barclay's fire escape garden in House Beautiful

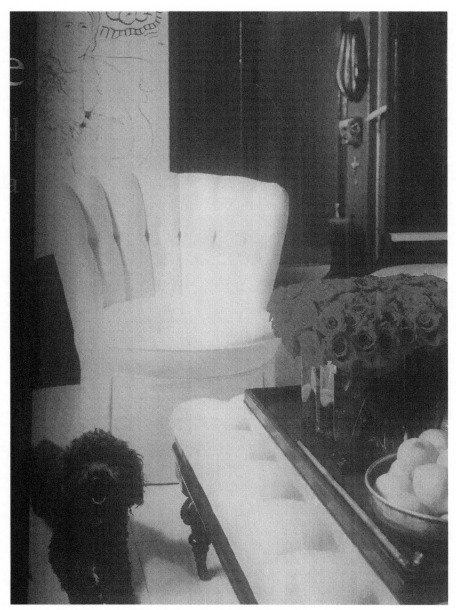

Mr. Pooh showing off his fabulous digs in House Beautiful

STAR CLOUT IN 2004

"Auditioning, pruning, prepping, manager, publicist—the whole nine yards, because I was preparing to be the next big household name. The Vice Chairman from Bergdorf Goodman wanted me to have my own chain of stores. I didn't sign on for that because he was sleazy, but that was still a highpoint. I was asked to have 300 stores around the world."

EARNING GRATITUDE FROM CELEBRITY CLIENTS

"People saying thank you after all those years. All I ever wanted was for someone to say thank you at the end of a project," says Barclay. "People like Lara Spencer—working for her was a highpoint." They met at a party, went out all night, and he became fast friends with the TV star (*Good Morning America*, *The Insider*, *Antiques Roadshow*) and author (*I Brake for Yard Sales, Flea Market Fabulous: Designing Gorgeous Rooms with Vintage Treasures*). Barclay decorated her gorgeous home in Riverside, Connecticut.

Being in *House Beautiful's* Top 100 Designers List

"The first year they did it, my name wasn't on the list. I called Carolyn Sollis and like a little brat, I said, 'I guess I wasn't good enough!' The next year, I made the list. It was like a USA stamp of approval, like a beef certification; I'd been branded. There are 100 designers in Fairfield County and I was the only one on this list. It was the Hadley crew. He was like the dean of design. It was very exciting to be amongst them and be labeled officially as one of them. I must have called 7,500 people and told them! And I did it without the casting couch, and there is a lot of that. More than in Hollywood. I've been chased around sofas, chased around pianos!" Barclay stayed on the list for close to a decade.

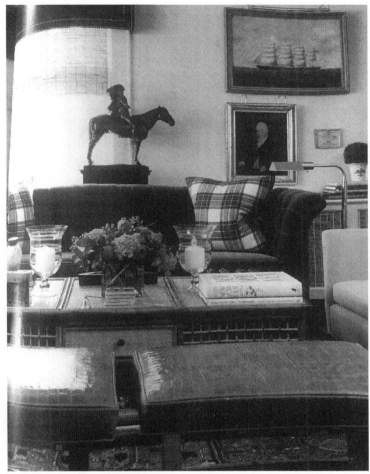

Lara Spencer's house in Riverside, CT, in Connecticut Cottages & Gardens *in 2005*

DOING DIANA ROSS'S AND LISA RINNA'S DRESSING ROOMS

"I did Diana Ross's dressing room as part of a charity concert at Greenwich Academy, selected from all the designers in Greenwich by the social ladies that I worked for. Bonnie Fuller asked to feature this project for *Celebrity Living* magazine. The dressing room, called 'Cool, Crisp, Chic,' was a dream. I had been in Diana's home before and knew her style. She loves purple. I used

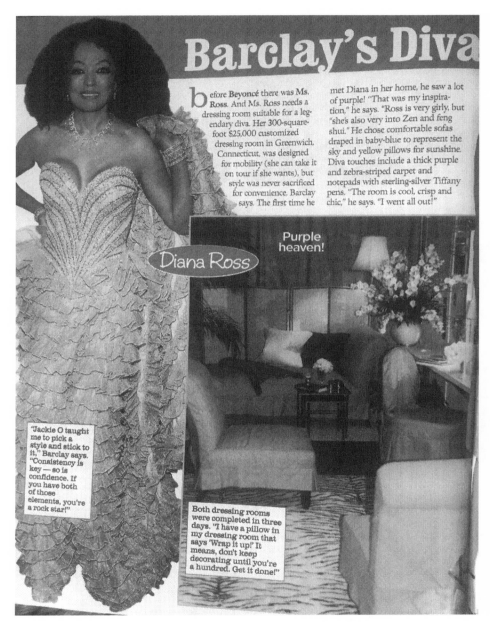

Barclay's Diva

before Beyoncé there was Ms. Ross. And Ms. Ross needs a dressing room suitable for a legendary diva. Her 300-square-foot $25,000 customized dressing room in Greenwich, Connecticut, was designed for mobility (she can take it on tour if she wants), but style was never sacrificed for convenience. Barclay says. The first time he met Diana in her home, he saw a lot of purple! "That was my inspiration," he says. "Ross is very girly, but "she's also very into Zen and feng shui." He chose comfortable sofas draped in baby-blue to represent the sky and yellow pillows for sunshine. Diva touches include a thick purple and zebra-striped carpet and notepads with sterling-silver Tiffany pens. "The room is cool, crisp and chic," he says. "I went all out!"

Diana Ross

Purple heaven!

"Jackie O taught me to pick a style and stick to it," Barclay says. "Consistency is key — so is confidence. If you have both of those elements, you're a rock star!"

Both dressing rooms were completed in three days. "I have a pillow in my dressing room that says 'Wrap it up!' It means, don't keep decorating until you're a hundred. Get it done!"

Diana Ross's and Lisa Rinna's dressing rooms in Celebrity Living *magazine*

Dressing Rooms

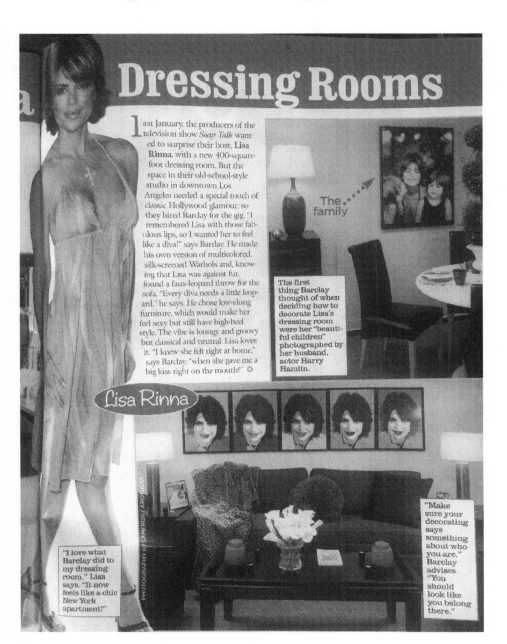

Last January, the producers of the television show *Soap Talk* wanted to surprise their host, **Lisa Rinna**, with a new 400-square-foot dressing room. But the space in their old-school-style studio in downtown Los Angeles needed a special touch of classic Hollywood glamour, so they hired Barclay for the gig. "I remembered Lisa with those fabulous lips, so I wanted her to feel like a diva!" says Barclay. He made his own version of multicolored, silk-screened Warhols and, knowing that Lisa was against fur, found a faux-leopard throw for the sofa. "Every diva needs a little leopard," he says. He chose low-slung furniture, which would make her feel sexy but still have high-heel style. The vibe is loungy and groovy but classical and neutral. Lisa loves it. "I knew she felt right at home," says Barclay, "when she gave me a big kiss right on the mouth!" ✪

The family

The first thing Barclay thought of when deciding how to decorate Lisa's dressing room were her "beautiful children" photographed by her husband, actor Harry Hamlin.

Lisa Rinna

"I love what Barclay did to my dressing room," Lisa says. "It now feels like a chic New York apartment!"

"Make sure your decorating says something about who you are," Barclay advises. "You should look like you belong there."

PHOTOGRAPHY BY CAMERON CAROTHERS

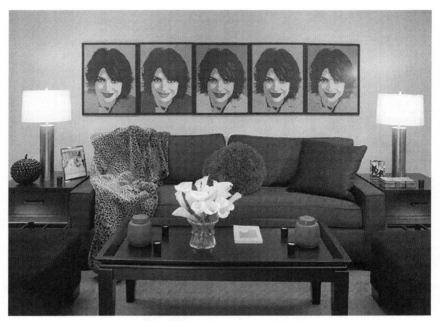

The "Barclay-hols" Barclay created for Lisa Rinna

baby blue, yellow, and purple. She owned one of the original Warhol pink Marilyns. I found another one and borrowed it from a client to use in the dressing room. I had fish swimming in vases with floating candles. I had custom carpets and curtains made. I spent two or three days to make sure it was perfect.

"Lisa Rinna, from *Housewives of Beverly Hills*, was a joy. She was hosting *Soap Talk* at the time. In the Warhol manner, I took a picture of her and made what I called Barclay-hols—my version of Andy Warhol's portraits. I put six of them over the sofa of her—lips and all. She was so excited to be honored that way. I made monogrammed napkins. I had custom sofas and chairs made *overnight*. I pulled out all the stops. When Lisa saw the room, she ran and jumped in my arms and kissed me with those lips." Barclay chuckles as he says, "It scared the hell out of me."

BEING ON THE COVER OF *GREENWICH MAGAZINE* IN 2005

"I passed the Moffly test—my goodness! It was exciting. I felt like I'd arrived finally in Greenwich. You almost have to be published nationally before you are published locally in *Greenwich* magazine. The picture was drop-dead fabulous because I was so proud and that showed through. Then *Stamford Advocate Weekly*, a Hearst publication, did a 10-page feature on me. I felt like I'd arrived in Fairfield County."

WORKING WITH A&E

"One winter morning I walked out of my building in Greenwich and there was a film crew milling around on the sidewalk. They were lost, hungry, and tired. No one would speak with them about the Skakle murder, but I would. I invited them up to my apartment, and before I even spoke a word I called and asked other friends to open their doors to them. Before long they had all the interviews they needed for the story. That day was the beginning of a 10-year relationship.

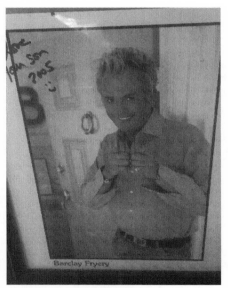

Barclay's Headshot in 2005, signed "Love Your Son"

They began to book me on *Biography; City Confidential;* and *Mansions, Monuments & Masterpieces*, which was a vehicle tailored for me, among other shows. I was a talking head on 50 or 60 shows, including *Style Court* on the Style Network. It was a lot of bad hair and too much makeup—rouge overload!—but it was fun. I was one of the top guys to audition for *Trading Spaces*, but I was too qualified; I was too expensive for them. I was also one of the top auditionees for *Queer Eye for the Straight Guy*. In the end, I would not take the role because 'queer' was in the title. For a while I was doing TV, print, and a radio show—*Barclay & Devora*—all at same time."

Shooting *Moochers* With Dr. Phil for CBS

"I really got hooked on television. This show was a vehicle to see if Jay McGraw (Dr. Phil's son) could handle millions of dollars in budget and it was the precursor to *The Doctors*. It did not end up airing. If it had, on this major network, it would have made me a household name. I was devastated, but it was a wonderful experience."

For a guy who struggled for acceptance growing up, the social highlights are dizzying:

"Meeting **Oscar Larrat**. He became *thee* top designer in Paris and my best, best friend in the world. I have one of his paintings in my living room. He's now famous. We had such fun together in Paris. We went to black-tie parties on motorcycles. We piled six people into a Mini, not the new Minis, an old Mini! He gave a dinner party in his bedroom for 40 people at one long table, in my honor. And there were prostitutes, models, princesses, train stewards—everyone was there. I said, 'You can't pull that off!' He said, 'Look behind the door,' where he had the boards for the table. And we all sat on cushions. He served pasta and a salad and wine. It was absolutely fabulous. He is really a chic guy.

"Being friends with **Cece Guest**, **Susie Hilfiger** (Tommy's first wife), **Letitia Baldrige**. Meeting **Marian McEvoy**, my first interior design editor. Meeting *Tear Sheet* magazine investor Paul Womack in Paris and having him tell me, 'You have style. You can write about fashion in Paris for us,' and then meeting you. All those parties in New York, in my Upper East Side crowd. Being treated like a human being after being treated so badly as a child. Being friends with **Fergie**, through an AIDS foundation. Meeting **Glenn Close** several times—she's so fabulous and sweet!

"Being at a bar, tapping on someone's shoulder, and saying, 'You look like **Fran Lebowitz**.' To which she responds in that deep voice, 'I am.' And then we spent the whole weekend hanging out with the rock-n-roll critic Lisa Robinson, crawling in the stacks in bookstores looking for books. Inviting her to dinner at Antoine's, and she walks in in cowboy boots, men's jeans, a striped Brooks Brothers shirt, and a blue blazer. Lee Radziwill had just been turned away in a Givenchy pantsuit. I said, 'How did you get past the door?' She replied, 'Their eyes never left mine.' It's all confidence. That was fabulous.

"Writing my column, *Ask Barclay*, every week in the *Greenwich Post*. I loved it. I started with Q&A and then added a little sidebar called 'Fresh Observations.' Most editors want columnists just to do Q&A. The day 'Fresh Observations' took over the whole column— that was a highpoint. My observations were respected. I reported on what was hot in theater, at parties. It wasn't a gossip column; it was a lifestyle column, on how to live life to the fullest. This was before lifestyle was really big. My editor, Doug Miller, liked me so much he let me do it. He understood the frustration of people being put in a box, and I tried to live outside the box my entire life. I also loved writing about **Oleg Cassini** for *Tear Sheet* magazine. I wanted to meet him so I pitched that story.

"I was a superstar for 15 years, until the recession. I traveled to Europe, shopping and exploring. I went to Vienna; Marrakech; Fez; Tangier; Paris, of course, my favorite place; London; St. Tropez; Ibiza. I got an education through travel and meeting people, and having fun and indulging just enough. I made great friends

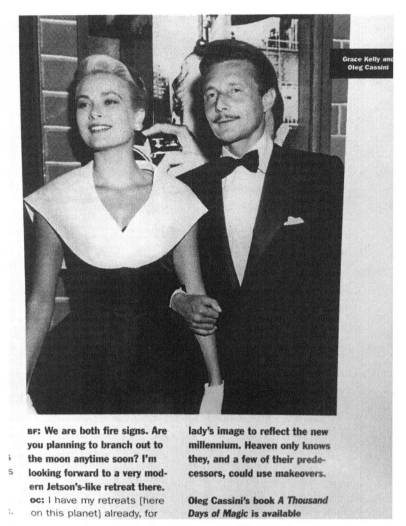

Grace Kelly and
Oleg Cassini

BF: We are both fire signs. Are you planning to branch out to the moon anytime soon? I'm looking forward to a very modern Jetson's-like retreat there.
OC: I have my retreats [here on this planet] already, for lady's image to reflect the new millennium. Heaven only knows they, and a few of their predecessors, could use makeovers.

Oleg Cassini's book *A Thousand Days of Magic* **is available**

Oleg Cassini and Grace Kelly in Barclay's article, "The Big O," in Tear Sheet *magazine*

in Paris and styled many apartments there. I shared an apartment in Paris with a close friend, and it became my post to then go out into the world. I did the European thing, the North African thing, the chic beach thing, the Nantucket thing. But Greenwich still drew me.

"I love Greenwich. Instead of New York City, I went to Greenwich. It had trees. It had the right clientele. It had the ocean and a simpler life that was not so busy as the city. It was wonderful. I began to speak to people on the sidewalk—'hello, good morning, hello'—and people started to speak! It's crazy how one or two people can be friendly and the whole town started to be friendly. I've been called a Greenwich icon—I don't know if that is true, but when I left Greenwich after 21 years, I left part of my soul there. It's where I made all my lasting adult friendships. It's where I did my best work. It's where people didn't judge me, where people accepted me for being a fabulous creature—which I of course had created, but weren't we all in caves at one time?"

> *"I've been called a Greenwich icon—I don't know if that is true, but when I left Greenwich after 21 years, I left part of my soul there."*

Barclay encourages me to call Wendie Force, one of his friends from that era. "I met him through his column 20 years ago," says Wendie, who is warm and eager to talk. "I was having trouble figuring out how to decorate my living room. I wrote a letter to him, and he gave me some advice and some designer names. I just needed a couple of rooms done. I called the designers, and you know how Greenwich prices are, they said, 'We usually do the whole house, but we could probably help you out for $75,000.'" Barclay agreed to help Wendie, at a reasonable rate.

"He came in with a sketchbook," says Wendie. "That's the way he works. It's all in his head, not in fancy computer programs." Barclay devised a grand plan, which included doing Wendie's living room in red and gold. She thought he was nuts: "I said, 'Red and

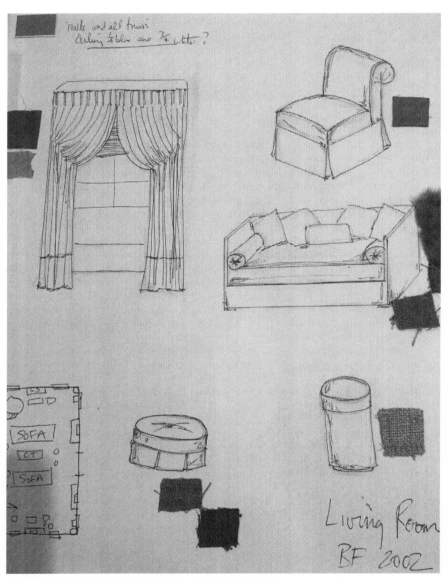

Samples of sketches from Barclay's design sketchbook

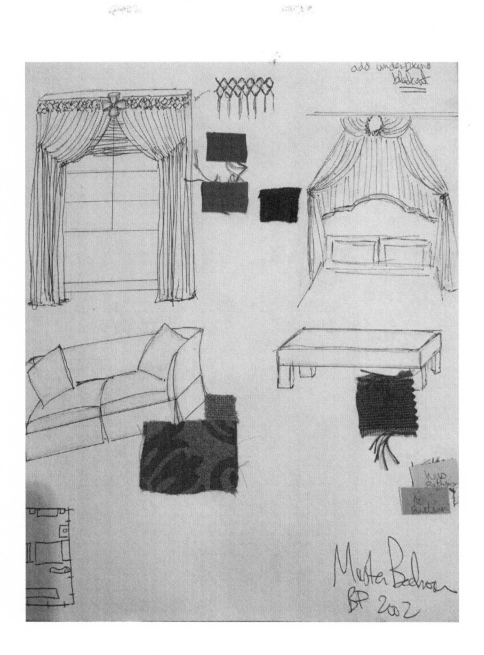

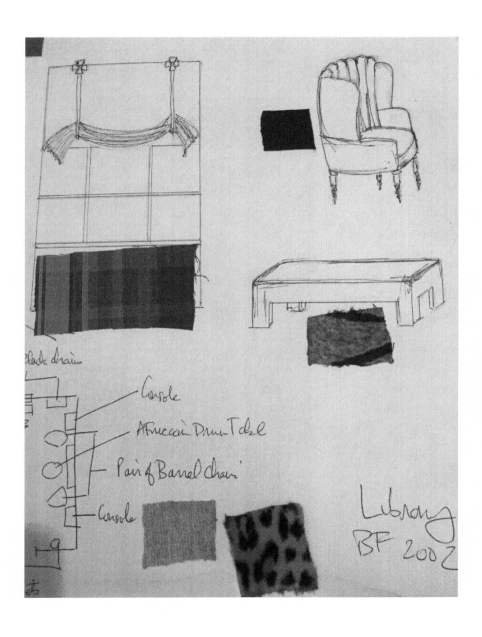

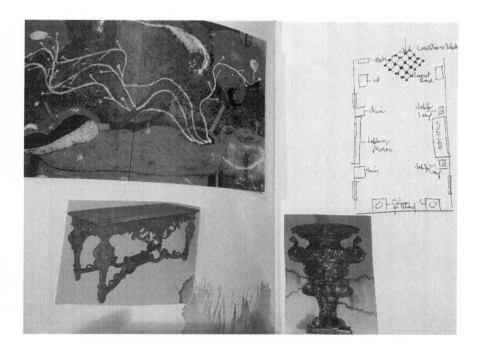

gold? No!' It was not what I had envisioned. I came from the era of all white. He told me, 'You are regal. This is right for you.' He was right. It looks amazing.

"Barclay had the couches and sectionals custom made, which turned out to be cheaper than going to Bloomie's. I'd see a sectional there that I really liked and drag Barclay to see it. He'd take one look and say, 'Wendie, *no!*'"

That was two decades ago, and Wendie hasn't changed any of Barclay's decor. "I look at that living room and it puts a smile on my face every day," she says.

Wendie was a single mom with a young boy when she first met Barclay. "There were Fisher Price toys all over my house then," comments Wendie. "Barclay got to know my son, Jordan. We became friends. Then he contacted me because he needed some smaller spaces for his portfolio. He did my son's room at cost. It ran in *House Beautiful*. He sneakily took all those awful 'before' pictures when I was moving stuff out of the room. The first time I saw them was in the magazine!

"I remember the three of us going to look for furniture at the mall. We went into Crate and Barrel, and I left them while I did an errand. I came back and the two of them were sitting in this gigantic sleigh bed. Barclay yelled, 'This is perfect!' I said, 'Barclay, his room is 12 x 15! He won't have any floor space.'" Accustomed to working in mansions, Barclay had to adjust the scale. They settled on a twin sleigh bed. Wendie chuckles as she says, "Barclay insisted on putting a *white* comforter on it. I said, 'Barclay, my son is 14!' We've managed it, just barely!"

Only Barclay, the optimist, would match white with a teenage boy. But the man with the closet full of snowy white shirts put his faith in the kid, and so the stains were kept at bay. While Barclay's design aesthetic is clean, Wendie confides that some of the ditties in her collection of Barclay Fryery Morning Voice Mails are too

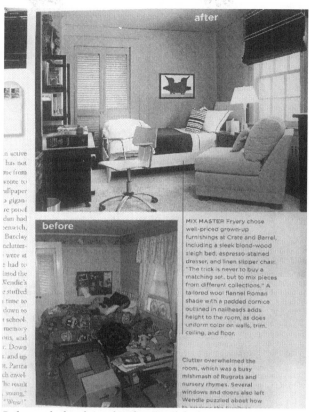

Before and after shots of Jordan Force's bedroom, in
House Beautiful

dirty for her to repeat from her desk at work! "They were very, very funny," she says. "He never said his name, but I always knew it was him."

"I've left her naughty ones and playful ones—like a Thanksgiving one of me gobbling like a turkey—and more *naughty* ones," recalls Barclay, with a chuckle.

When Barclay was in Greenwich last year, Wendie hired him to do a consultation on her upstairs. "When I talked to him recently, I told him I'm so happy he's doing this book. I said, 'Barclay, I want a signed copy, and the color you picked for the spare bedroom is . . . kind of unusual. You can't die on me yet, because I don't know what to do with this! I'll have to go back to white, and you don't want me to do that."

BARCLAY DIRECTS ME TO A STACK OF magazines in his living room, including the *House Beautiful* that showcases the makeover of Jordan's room. There are about 30, and within each Barclay's design work appears, or he is featured, or he has written an article. A small, spiral-bound lookbook with an elegant logo showcases the Barclay Fryery Collection, his furniture line, which debuted in 2005. "I made each piece couture, for each client," says Barclay, whose favorite piece is the Day Bed. "I have one in leopard in my living room. It's low-slung and sexy." Much of the furniture in his apartment comes from the line.

House Beautiful *describes Barclay's style as:* "simple, hip, alive."

Spread after spread features Barclay's work—from American Federal farmhouses to modern makeovers, decadent projects to low-budget magic, and groovy rooms mixed with classic touches, like an 18th-century French bust in his funky bathroom. There's Lara Spencer's Riverside carriage house and Diana Ross's dressing room—each decorated flawlessly, to reflect the distinct style of each client.

House Beautiful describes Barclay's style as: "simple, hip, alive." *Alive.* It's an adjective that will live on as the brand Barclay Fryery endures, even after the person is gone. Those who love Barclay might take a tip from him on coping with the inevitable: compartmentalize. Timothy Mark will be gone, gone to live with the angels. Barclay Fryery will live on.

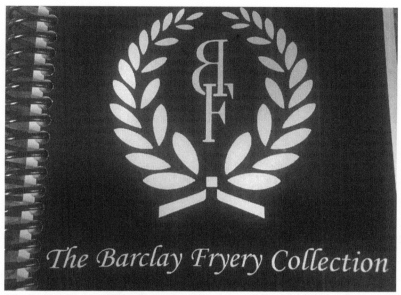

The Barclay Fryery Collection Lookbook

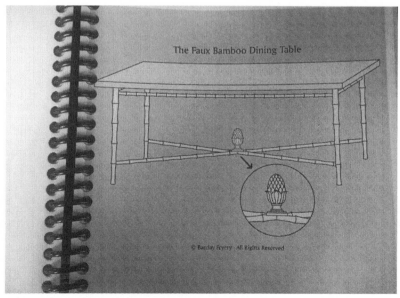

The Bamboo Table from the Barclay Fryery Collection

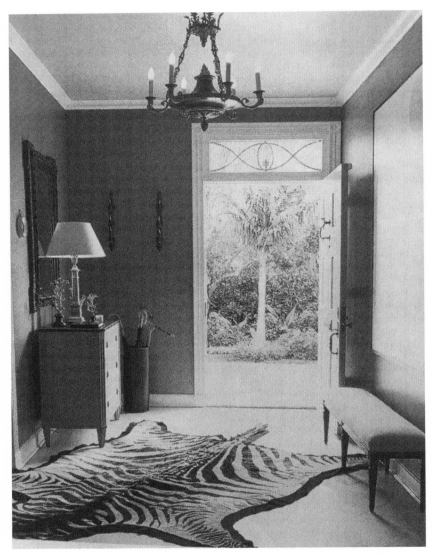

Mark Freitas, the owner of this Palm Beach mansion, says he's never seen a Fryery project that he hasn't admired. Featured in Palm Beach Cottages & Gardens, *2005*

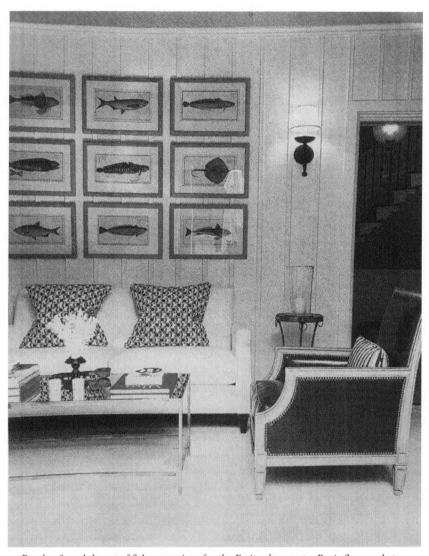

Barclay found the set of fish engravings for the Freitas home at a Paris flea market

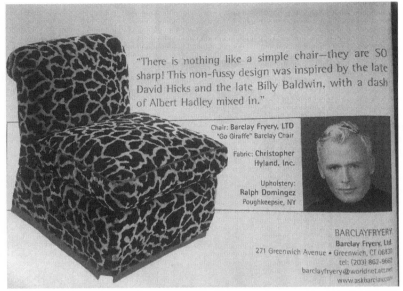

"There is nothing like a simple chair—they are SO sharp! This non-fussy design was inspired by the late David Hicks and the late Billy Baldwin, with a dash of Albert Hadley mixed in."

Chair: Barclay Fryery, LTD
"Go Giraffe" Barclay Chair

Fabric: Christopher Hyland, Inc.

Upholstery:
Ralph Domingez
Poughkeepsie, NY

BARCLAYFRYERY
Barclay Fryery, Ltd
271 Greenwich Avenue • Greenwich, CT 06830
tel: (203) 862-9662
barclayfryery@worldnet.att.net
www.askbarclay.com

The Barclay Chair, in House Beautiful *in 2003*

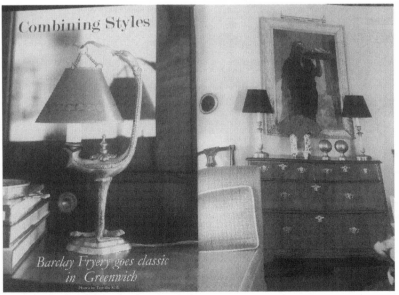

Combining Styles

Barclay Fryery goes classic in Greenwich

American Federal style in Fairfield County Home

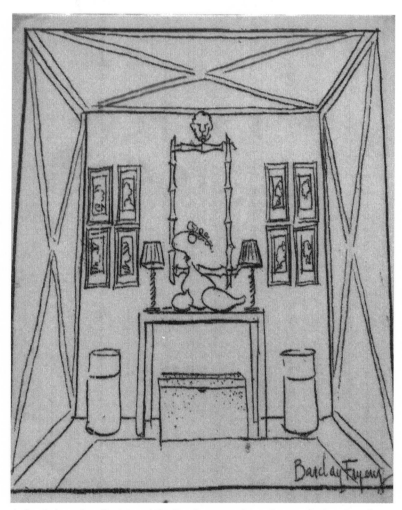

A sketch from the all-white exhibit Barclay created in tribute to the late David Hicks, at the Southport Garden Festival with Albert Hadley

Enjoy decorating tips, articles, tear sheets, and videos from Barclay in the "Design" section on: CancerLooksGoodonYou.com

CHAPTER 5

Angels

—◦—◦—◦—◦—◦—

Kindness, Facebook, and Barclay's Angels—
Lessons in Compassion and Connection

"ANGELS" IS THE TERM BARCLAY applies to all the helpful people swirling around him in life. Every one of them sets an example for how to behave when someone is in need. Barclay's kind heart and generous spirit naturally have attracted benevolent folks along his path—this is the logical explanation and lesson to live by. He is a model for good karma.

However, in Barclay's eyes, angels have been *sent* to him. An entire brigade of angels swooped in to carry him through cancer. Barclay faced his demons and diseases with courage, clawed at them with unassailable optimism, and staved off the ugly side of everything with a laser focus on beauty. But he is insistent that he could not have done it without benevolent attendants along the way—seemingly sent to him by a God who wanted to make up for all the mixed messages Barclay received about the fate of his soul.

Born into a household in which "everything was a sin," Barclay desperately needed a guardian angel when he was a boy. She came in the form of the baby sister he'd wished for on Santa's knee. As the older brother, Barclay was Lisa's protector more than she was his, but that gave him purpose. "I paved the way for her as we got older, so she wouldn't have the troubles I had," says Barclay. "I made sure she fit in. I made sure she got in the right sorority." When Barclay considered suicide as a teen, he could not go through with it because he could not crush his angelic mother or squash his angel Bug. As a gay boy in a strict Evangelical family, he also knew he would not see these dear angels again if he ended his life, because he would go to hell.

Despite the harsh lessons conveyed at church, some angels came to Barclay from there as well. "The preacher's daughter, Susan Frazier, snuck me to my first big audition," says Barclay. Without her, he would not have landed his wise Owl role and perhaps none of the other empowering roles would have followed. Years later it was Susan's mom, Dot, the preacher's wife, who comforted Barclay after the horrible garbage lid beating from his father. She held his hand and sent the message that he would overcome, and he did—both on the stage that night and in life.

Barclay remembers his pediatrician, Dr. McEachin reaching out as well. "He noticed some welts on me and asked me what was going on, so I told him," recalls Barclay. "He took me under his arm and led me to Central Methodist, where there was a big youth group, and I could escape from what I was going through. Had he not done that, I don't know where I would have been. Then I evolved to the Episcopalian church, but I was a Methodist for a very long time.

"When I was 15, another angel was sent to me: Sonja DiMeola. She was a rebel in my French class. Junior year, the school's annual and newspaper staff went to New York. I craved to go but didn't have the money. So she hired me as her driver in high school and paid me to take her to and from school. That's how I afforded the trip. In New York, I saw big things, bold things, scary things . . . I got lost in Harlem in a snowstorm. I was frightened as all get-out, but it opened my eyes. Had it not been for Sonja, I would not have seen New York! Any way I found to escape, in a positive way, I did—whether through magazines, or auditions, or going to New York. But without these players, I would have faced only roadblocks."

"Any way I found to escape, in a positive way, I did."

Barclay also could not imagine his path had he not met several men who guided him in understanding and accepting his sexuality. There was Daniel, in college, who groomed Barclay as a coming-of-age gay man, modeling confidence and bravado and bronzer! "Whenever someone at school would get jealous of me, they would call my parents and say, 'You know, your son sucks dick.' I knew to go to Daniel and he would help me. He was so out in a time when people were so narrow-minded. I still apologize to him to this day for being so insecure."

Daniel continued to be Barclay's touchstone through the years. "He is mischievously clever, peppy, steadfast, and bursting with love," says Barclay. "His mom, Hazeline Harrington, loaned me money for my first down payment in New Orleans after rehab, to get me started again. She took my Louis Vuitton as hostage to make sure I paid her back! It was very cute. She was like the kind version of Cruella De Vil. Whenever they went broke, I'd send her a new

Kate Spade patent leather purse with a perfume, a wallet, and a little note for an unlimited lunch on me. I flew Daniel to Greenwich, to Palm Beach, to New York, sent him Cartier watches and boots. They were good to me, and then when I had money, I was good to them. They are wonderful angels I was blessed to cross paths with. She died recently, sadly, so Daniel's kind of lost. He has been wonderful in every aspect of my life."

Barclay's next angel helped him understand that he would not be barred from reconnecting with his earthly angels up in heaven. "I met Michael Ronkese at Rehobeth Beach on a beautiful weekend in 1983. He had a beach house there," recalls Barclay. "We became instant friends because he was in the church, and I thought that's where I had to go for salvation. I mean, at this time I was still scalding myself in the shower every morning hoping to burn away the gay, so that I would be *normal.* That went on for a decade.

> *"I struck the priesthood off my bucket list and finally embraced who I was born to be, fully and without regret or guilt."*

"Michael was a priest. I had wanted to go into the priesthood to just disappear. I thought, due to my strict religious upbringing, that's what I needed to do to keep from going to hell. Michael convinced me otherwise since he had taken that path for the same reason. He was commissioned to be sent to the Vatican to be groomed for greatness, but he realized he would be throwing away his true self—who he was born to be—if he went. Instead, he left the priesthood.

"Needless to say, I struck the priesthood off my bucket list and finally embraced who I was born to be, fully and without regret or guilt. Thank you, Michael Ronkese! He was my guardian angel, for sure." Receiving the news that this dear friend was dying of AIDS and caring for him during his last days in DC left a hole in Barclay's heart, but it was a heart that was forever fortified by their relationship.

When Barclay faced his own HIV crisis, he again turned to a holy place. He found a gay priest and acceptance at Christ Church in Greenwich. "They got me off the ground, as all Episcopalian churches do," says Barclay. He always managed to sift through the dogma and find the people in the church who were there because they were caring, not judgmental. He could have been bitter and scoffed at religion and its doctrines, but it is like Barclay wears a pair of magical glasses that block out the bad and only let in the good. They are a nifty accessory we all should try. Bitterness, resentment—they have no place in Barclay's philosophy.

"ANGELS TRANSLATES FROM THE Hebrew to 'messengers sent by God,' which could be earthly people in your life that heaven sends to your path to guide and assist you in your time of need . . . I am so blessed daily!" (Facebook Post, April 7, 2017)

The social network has served as a psychological net, catching Barclay every time he falls into a fit of depression, exhaustion, or loneliness—states cancer has a way of eliciting on a regular basis.

Social media—we curse it more often than we praise it. But Facebook has been Barclay's saving grace for the last two years. The social network has served as a psychological net, catching Barclay every time he falls into a fit of depression, exhaustion, or loneliness—states cancer has a way of eliciting on a regular basis.

On Facebook, he has reconnected with past angels in his life and new ones have found him there.

I notice a card on Barclay's kitchen windowsill. The elegant panther in black and gold ink and the pretty cursive on the Cartier stationary catch my eye. It reads:

> *Dearest Barclay,*
> *May this little gift help to refresh your wellness. Surround you with comfort. Encircle you with healing, and remind you that you are not alone in this journey.*
>
> *I pray that you receive from God all the help you need. I pray that you are cradled in hope. Kept in joy. Graced with peace and wrapped in love always.*
>
> *Have a beautiful day my friend and if you ever need to talk, I'm a call away.*
> *With love,*
> *Lauren xo*

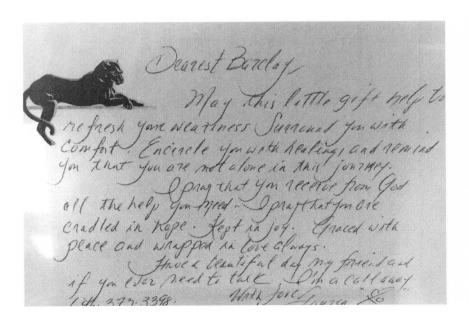

At a loss for words with someone suffering from a grave illness? My goodness, this notes says it all. Perfectly. I ask Barclay who this eloquent woman is. "Oh, that's from Lauren Laremore. She's a designer in Greenwich, a wonderful person," he says. "She calls me every morning and every night."

Lauren happens to call while I am there, so we chat a bit. "Barclay has a nice brigade of angels who look over him, and I'm honored to be one of them," she tells me. "He is ever present in my thoughts and prayers. I keep praying for a miracle and I do believe in miracles. I lost my husband to cancer. I know all too well what that road is like, the highs and lows. Cancer is a very lonely disease. When my husband got sick, our friends dropped off the face of the earth. People don't know what to do and say, so unfortunately they stay away. But it's the time when you really need the support of your friends. I'm sorry I can't be there with Barclay, but I try to keep up with him on a daily basis. I'm blessed to have healthy children. My heart goes out to a young man like Barclay, who is suffering and going through such a hard time."

I ask Lauren how she met Barclay. I figure they must be long-time Greenwich pals. "We've known each other our whole lives, but we've never met," she says. "You could say we are soulmates. I began following his journey on Facebook two years ago. I was drawn to his lovely posts. He painted such beautiful pictures with his words. I started liking his posts. I started giving him little words of encouragement. I let him know he is being worried about."

Their story gives new meaning to finding long lost family members on Facebook. Lauren has become a mother figure to Barclay, filling in for those phone calls Barclay can no longer have with his own mom. "The Italian mother comes out in me," continues Lauren, "I'm always asking Barclay, 'Have you eaten? Are you hydrated?'"

Barclay adds, "Sometimes her 'Brooklyn girl' comes out too.

Last year, I reconnected with a friend from Ole Miss. I taught her to swing dance at her dorm 30 years ago. We had spent only a half-hour together, but when we happened to be at the same nail salon in Meridian getting pedicures, she recognized my voice. She asked, 'Are you Fryery?' She asked me to come see her place in Decatur and asked me if I'd escort her to parties, as her husband was often unavailable. For Christmas she sent me a gift certificate for the same mani-pedi spa, but the ownership had changed. They told me, 'No serve men!' They were very rude and wouldn't give me a refund, either.

"Lauren called and we were chitchatting and I told her what happened. She immediately got on the phone with the state board and complained about the nail salon. She told me, 'I may be in Greenwich now, but I'm from Brooklyn!'" The salon got slapped with a fine.

He lost a pedicure. He gained the courage to start revealing parts of his story that felt painful or shameful before.

"I had just been on the news in an HIV story, so maybe that's why they wouldn't serve me," ponders Barclay, "but you can't catch it that way! Amicia Ramsey, a reporter who lives next door, did a story on life with HIV and I was the feature. I've never told the truth about that. I've always hidden it. But I decided, what do I have to lose?" He lost a pedicure. He gained the courage to start revealing parts of his story that felt painful or shameful before. If Barclay hadn't already earned his wings, this is the moment where that little bell in *It's a Wonderful Life* rings and he becomes an angel to so many people who are as lost and scared as he once was.

One Facebook follower, a young transgender man named

Hank Doyle, writes: "Knowing you, even peripherally, has made my life infinitely better. Thank you."

"Every day my friend Barclay Fryery is alive, it's a gift to all of us and a lesson in how to behave when life gets difficult."

Candice Valentine posts: "We have friends and then we have friends that touch your heart for life. Every day my friend Barclay Fryery is alive, it's a gift to all of us and a lesson in how to behave when life gets difficult. His fight and his genteel way of giving us all life each day is everything. He is one of God's angels on Earth and I feel blessed that I'm a part of his magical life. Thank you sweet Barclay for showing me so many much-needed lessons in life. I adore you." Candice refers to Barclay as her "cyber husband." They have never met.

Jane Coco Cowles is ever-present in Barclay's newsfeed, encouraging him and offering support. "He is one of the most interesting, fun, and kind-hearted people I know," comments Jane. Barclay says, "I met Jane at Richards years ago. Now she's an artist. She sends me surprises every week, cards stuffed with cash, and donates to my GoFundMe. We have become great friends through this journey." She puts him and this book perfectly into a nutshell when she posts: "Barclay Fryery, the man known for his 'Ask Barclay' column, fabulous style, and sometimes naughty sense of humor . . . walks through cancer with grace. *Cancer Looks Good on You* Tells All."

AFTER BARCLAY ANNOUNCES ON Facebook that he starts hospice care on March 29, 2017, a chorus of commenters responds instantly with sympathy, memories, gratitude, praise.

Bruce McIntosh writes: "You expressing your journey on Facebook I'm sure is extremely difficult. But what you are doing is probably the most important thing you've done in your life. Your inspiration is truly magnificent Barclay. Thank you for your courage, as I have spent my time in a hospice too and your kindness is really appreciated."

He found himself on a pedestal in a town where he grew up feeling like he was in the gutter.

Marianne Walters Todd recalls: "I will never forget photographing you leading a packed house at the Riley Center. And they were all there to see YOU, to hang on your every word, each hoping to walk away with a fraction of your knowledge and talent!" She reminds him of that highlight, when he found himself on a pedestal in a town where he grew up feeling like he was in the gutter. Imagine!

Nicole Facciuto posts: "In 2003 I was cast in my first design show, *House Wars*. Sitting next to me in first class was a vibrant human being, who would come to be my friend and also design rival on the show. I shared with him how to use tape to create dimension with paint, as he was dumbfounded on how to work with a small $10K budget per room. He has worked design magic for so many high-end residences in New York, Connecticut, and beyond. He is quite possibly in his final week of life on this planet. Barclay Fryery, you are a wonder and a delight. What an honor and joy it has been to hear your voice and laughter over the 14 years I've known you. You've touched so many of our hearts and spirits."

From Carol Brodie: "Barclay, I hope that you are somehow in peace. Beautiful souls fly with angels always."

Barclay posts about the nurses who are helping him through: "My nurse Louise, another angel from heaven, is on her way to sort my multitude of meds that I can no longer take care of since I see double due to the morphine levels that are necessary to keep me ahead of the enormous pains of having cancer all over my body! I could not survive without your kindness, help and support! Thank you!"

Another time he writes, "I could not survive without my daily hospice angel Crystal. She enables me to bathe and dress in a civilized manner during this difficult journey of cancer. She puts the laundry on after the bath and folds yesterday's. I could never have the strength to do that. A little mothering helps this old boy get through his day! God bless you."

THERE ARE ANGELS, AND THEN THERE are *Barclay's Angels*: "Choo," Renae, and Kate. I like to picture them in a *Charlie's Angels* pose, surrounding Barclay in his bedroom slipper chair. In place of guns and karate-chop hands would be lattes and pillow-fluffing action. To understand the timeliness of this celestial trio's arrival on the scene, let's go back to the Great Recession.

The financial crisis that hit in 2008 marked a turning point for Barclay. The *Moochers* pilot didn't air, another show Barclay had landed for the *Style* network fell through, and clients began defaulting on payments. Barclay, once a millionaire, saw his savings dwindling. He fell into a depression and turned to food for comfort. Before long, Barclay was almost bankrupt, 140 pounds heavier, and had nowhere to turn but back.

"Moving back to Meridian was real hard," says Barclay. "I slept for a year and a half, pretty much. It was my *Egoiste* Period. Millions were affected by the recession, but in my mind it was only me. It was pride. From 2011 to 2013, I lived in my sister's cottage on her farm. I knew no one except high school friends, who now have grandchildren. It was more rural than I remembered. I was lost back here. But once I stopped blaming people for my problems and took responsibility for some bad decisions, I started to come out of my shell."

Barclay ran into an old classmate, Adele Williamson Graham, at his sister's antique store. "She was an heiress, the prettiest girl in school, and wild as a March hare," recounts Barclay. "I was wary of her but this was a new, glowing, angel version of Adele." (Another angel. They seem to keep sneaking into the story!)

Adele shared her recollection of the encounter: "We hadn't seen each other since high school and when we laid eyes on one another, Barclay screamed with delight, 'Oh my, you're Adele . . . WOOOWWWW.' We instantly reconnected. Of course I wanted to call him Tim but was quickly reprimanded and told he should always be addressed as Barclay. 'Sweetie, call me Barclay,' he insisted. That took a little time to get used to yet Barclay he was! He was very different from the kid I remembered in high school. I was very different too. I was recovering from substance abuse, and Barclay was recovering from his financial fall in Connecticut. We were both a little broken. We clicked."

Barclay says, "Adele had found sobriety and was running a center and retreat for others recovering from drugs and alcohol, called TAME." They became fast friends and found common ground between his misery from losing everything and hers from having too much. "I cried many a day about the past with her and what was," says Barclay, "and she reminded me to let it go. We ate almost every meal together, and she made me an honorary Williamson for every holiday."

Adele recalls, "One day in 2012, Barclay burst through the door and trapped me in the kitchen. He was singing and I was laughing, when suddenly he got down on one knee and proposed marriage! Not your typical marriage, mind you, but a proposal nonetheless. I accepted and we became inseparable. Barclay helped me design TAME, my home, and many of my friends' and relatives' homes—all with his usual flare and quirkiness. My family welcomed him with open arms."

"Suddenly he got down on one knee and proposed marriage!"

Barclay says, "I was the gay husband. She really was the catalyst that brought me back from the abyss. She is also six foot four and blond! She's very funny and always laughing and smiling. We danced down the aisles at Winn Dixie, using our grocery carts as walkers." Adele adds, "We would push our carts while holding all sorts of kooky poses, as we sang through the aisles to the elevator music. I literally would laugh so hard that I had tears streaming down my face!"

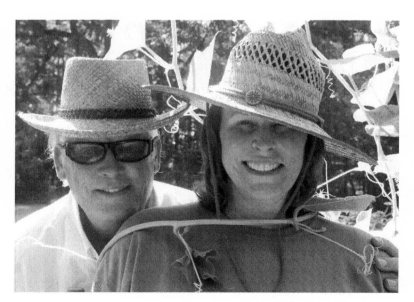

Barclay also found his way to St. Paul's Episcopal Church. "Again the Episcopal church," says Barclay. "And there were stylish people, chic people, people who had teeth in their mouths, you know! Through that I began to do some work. I was longing to go back to New York, but then I realized you can't get that twice. Very few get it once. To reclaim that, that big life . . . It was exhausting, the thought of it. I was not young anymore. I was not fresh. Then lo and behold, I get a lump in the side of my neck, and I have cancer.

> *I believe that period of dwelling on my problems—that uber sadness, doubt, and fear—had caused the cancer to fester.*

"I was *de-va-stated*. How, after all I'd done and all I'd been through, how could that happen to me? I believe that period of dwelling on my problems—that uber sadness, doubt, and fear— had caused the cancer to fester.

"A client owed me a lot of money that they hadn't paid. And so a country club bill comes, and I couldn't pay it. Eventually I was thrown out of the club. I was sick and my career had stopped again. I saw doctors all over Meridian. I went to Jackson for a second opinion." In January of 2016, Barclay was told he had stage 4 cancer and seven months to live. He recalls feeling dumbfounded, thinking, *How is that possible; I have only seven months to live?*

Barclay found himself in an impossible position: he could not pay his bills or afford care, but people assumed he was rich. "I set up a GoFundMe account," says Barclay, "but there were naysayers everywhere. They were saying, 'Why is *he* asking for money?'"

How is that possible; I have only seven months to live?

But whatever deity or karmic force doles out angels to good people was not sleeping on the job—especially with the way Barclay has of coaxing angels from the universe. "People I would not ordinarily run with became my closest and dearest friends," says Barclay, "because they were real. Many of my rich, powerful friends walked away. I was shocked. People who could write a check and raise my $50,000 in a minute turned their back. The workingmen and women that were kind, responsible, 'normal' people all helped. Sometimes when they couldn't afford to, they still helped. Without the middle, I don't know where I would have been, and that's where I came from."

Barclay heard about Renae Gardner through an architect friend and hired her to paint his ceilings. "I explained how I wanted the banding, and she said, 'Ohhhhh, I can't do that.' I told her, 'You most certainly can!' When you believe in someone, they start believing in themselves. Mama always said, 'Can't never could do nothing!' Now, three years later, Renae is my best friend down here and one of the three angels who takes care of me."

From Renae's perspective, a design god has been sent to her. She has soaked in Barclay's expertise. "He always encourages, never lets anyone sell themselves short," says Renae, whose meticulous handiwork—the banding on the ceiling, the doors, the blades of an old ceiling fan glamorized with a coat the same color as the banding—keeps Barclay's apartment looking magazine-spread ready.

"I asked for help with my house, so we bartered," continues Renae. "He likes things very fresh. He could probably employ a full-time painter! I love just sitting in that chair across from him, learning all of his design intricacies. He introduced me to the

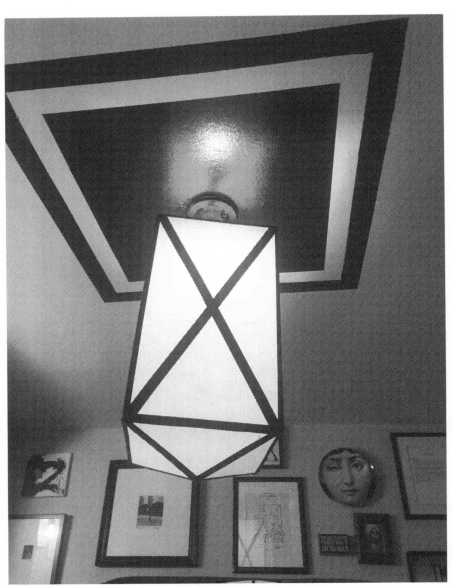

Renae's handiwork on Barclay's ceiling

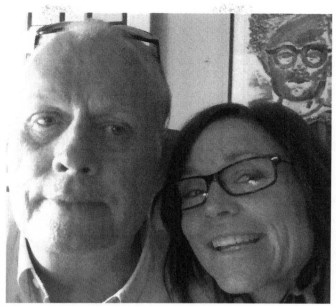

Barclay and Renae Gardner

concept of painting trim, molding, doors, and baseboards all the same shade but in different sheens."

Barclay chimes in, "Mr. Hadley taught me that. I just passed it on!"

Renae adds, "He'll look at pictures of homes I'm working on and advise on the design, saying move this here or this over there. He helps me pick colors. With built-in bookcases, he taught me to paint the back wall of the bookcase a different color to add dimension. Now he's trained me well enough that when I ask his opinion, I get a lot more, 'Yes, please's,' and not as many [imitating his velvety, deep voice] 'noooooooooooo!'s'"

Barclay does not have money to pay for care, but he has knowledge to share. Nobody feels like a burden in the relationship.

Renae, like everyone who knows Barclay, is in awe of his positive influence on all who cross his path. "He had to have a Ralph Lauren bracelet worked on at the shoe repair shop, so I dropped it off," she recounts. "The people there were really concerned about him. The cobbler told me how the first time Barclay came in, he wanted his Gucci Loafers repaired. He told Barclay, 'I don't know if I can do it.'"

Barclay explains, "He pushed the shoes back to me and I pushed them right back to him and said, 'I believe in you.' I named him Kenny the Cobbler."

Renae adds, "He was very worried about you." To which Barclay replies, "He's a lovely man."

Kate Cherry also stars as one of Barclay's Angels. "Kate is the Director of the Meridian Museum of Art and is hosting my after-party celebration. She stops by every day and makes sure I have eaten, even takes out the garbage. My first concern after diagnosis was what would happen to my babies. In steps Kate and voilà, all worry was lifted. She is a heavenly creative force and we have a special love fest going on. Kate is in many ways the most important cog in the exit plan because she is the new foster mom. She has already adopted Mr. Pooh and will also take The Princess Royale when I expire . . . keeping the family together," says Barclay, relieved.

"I had met Kate on several occasions, but I was in a fog most of the time then, missing New York, feeling displaced. I was trying to learn my hometown again, through my sister, who was a great help. Then when I did Darrah and Bill's wedding in the Bahamas in June, I was so happy there that I forgot about my cancer and laid out in the sun. I got a sunburn and it hit the radiation that was in my head and my neck, and I went cuckoo. I was literally *cuckoo*, for like two weeks. I called people at midnight not knowing why I was calling, and I was so sick.

"She opened her purse and laid $1,000 right here on my pink bench in one-hundred-dollar bills."

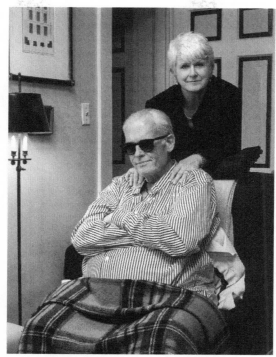

Barclay and Kate Cherry

"During that period, all of a sudden there is a knock on my door here in Meridian and in walks this glorious creature with white hair, the director of the Museum of Art. She sat down with me, and she saw my stress and the state of turmoil I was in. She opened her purse and laid $1,000 right here on my pink bench in one-hundred-dollar bills. She said, 'I know that you're distressed. Go pay your bills, so you don't get in trouble.' I thought, *Wow, that's nice*! It's something I would have done back when I could. It's not why we became friends. She had watched my career. She had the magazines I had been in. So then I offered to do her house for free. And that was the cottage I did out in Poplarville, where Mr. Pooh is now at home, with his new parents, Kate and Terry Cherry. She was sent to me.

"Of course the third Angel is Choo, Susie Womack Cannon, who just happened to look me up. I hadn't kept in touch with her. She was the young lady in the neighborhood my mother hand-picked to be our babysitter. I couldn't pronounce her name, so I called her 'Choo,' and I still do. Choo is here from 9 until 1 every day, making sure I have a hot meal and running all of my errands as if she is me. Those three people have surrounded me with love, support, comfort, spirituality, and kindness. Without these angels, I don't know how I would have made it."

When Barclay received his diagnosis, his second thought after thinking of his pets was: "Cancer is so ugly; how am I going to navigate through it?" With his angels by his side, Barclay found the answers. "I know it's strange to say," he adds, "but this has been the worst year of my life but also the best year of my life."

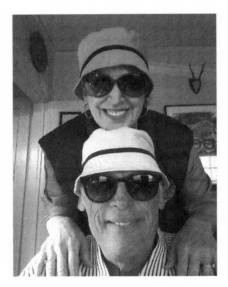

"It's a Ralph Lauren bucket hat celebration here at Hospice Fryery with yet another angel, but of the Arch-angel variety . . . here you will meet three! Meet Choo, aka Susie Womack Cannon, who rotates throughout

the week with Renae Gardner and Kate Cherry, also Archangels. They make sure Your Barclay has a hot meal when needed and errands taken care of . . . These gifts from the heavens are exactly just that GIFTS! Thank you, ladies."

(Facebook Post, April 6, 2017)

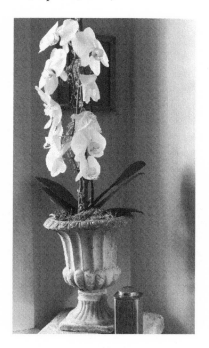

"I received the most exquisite white Phalaenopsis orchid, my all-time favorite, from World of Flowers . . . Thanks to one of my dearest, my angel Kate Cherry! God is in the details and the simplest thing can make your heart sing! I love you beyond words and appreciate all you do to keep me going day to day . . . Thank you!"

(Facebook Post, March 31, 2017)

CHAPTER 6

Closure

Making Amends, Planning a Funeral, Knowing When to "Wrap It Up"

"THOMAS WOLFE WROTE: 'You can't go home again.' I lived that," says Barclay. "But the silver lining through it all is multi-fold."

Barclay says he was able to "make amends with his father," though the reality is more complicated than that.

"Hate hurts you more than the person you are hating."

"In 2004, I had called my father and apologized for hating him all these years. I told him I really loved him and I asked for

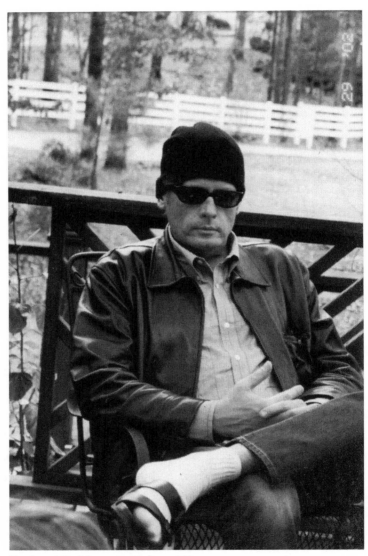

Barclay at Lisa's house in Madison, MS

his forgiveness. He didn't know what I was talking about. He had blocked it out. I asked for forgiveness, because hate hurts you. Hate hurts you more than the person you are hating.

"In the end, when he had dementia, I took care of my father. At the very end, I would get calls, at 2, 3, 4 in the morning, that he'd crawled or fallen out of bed. I'd go and clean his diaper, wipe the pee off him, prop chairs against the bed so he didn't climb out again. I'm not that strong anymore; this was only two years ago. I picked up this big man and tried to save his dignity."

Barclay's father knocked him to the ground. Barclay picked his father up off the ground. He struggled to find the strength, but the powerful message is clear.

"During that period, I was sitting on the sofa and he was by the fireplace. He asked me, 'You are my son, aren't you? I know that you are your mama's, but are you mine?'" Barclay replied, "Yes, I'm your son, Daddy."

"Then he asked me, 'You are married, aren't you?'" Barclay fibbed and said yes, and that his wife was living overseas in the foreign service. This pleased his father.

Barclay continues, "He told me, 'I didn't realize I'd like you as much as I like you.' At that instant all the hatred in my heart went away.

"The night before he died, I kissed him on the forehead. He snapped back and flinched, because boys don't do that. See, he was a wonderful man, but I just was not the typical son that he wanted. When he was in the coffin, I kissed him on the forehead again and fixed the monkey Hermes tie that I gave him to be buried in."

Later Barclay shares more with me. The stories are simmering below the surface, and it's clear he is still working his way to finding closure on this subject. "I sent him gifts throughout the years to try to buy his love: a Hermes jacket, ties, jodhpurs, shoes, boots, cologne. It was all really nice stuff. I treated him to the best I could afford. He once called and asked me for a car. I couldn't afford that at that time. I thought it was ballsy, after him treating me like *S-H-I-T* all my life."

I ask if he knows what his father's childhood was like.

"His father beat him, I've been told," he says. Barclay, the most gentle man of all gentlemen, stopped the cycle. He continues, "Abuse was normal to him. It's how he was brought up. He had five sisters—four half sisters and one real sister (the one who was raped at 12). My dad had to wear a dress until he was 12. It was a simple sack dress that was passed down—can you imagine?

"I believe his homophobia was expressed by him beating me. Hitler persecuted Jews and queers—he was both himself. I think my dad was a latent homosexual. He never acted on it."

Barclay insists I speak to several people about his father, to be sure he is portrayed fairly.

Aunt Evelyn, Barclay's mother's oldest sister, is the aunt who reprimanded Lee for giving Barclay a licking at her house. At 85, she sounds just as strong-minded now as she was then. "They were real ugly to Tim [Barclay], so ugly that I quit going to see them. I couldn't take it any longer," she says. "If I been Frances, he would have only done that but one time. I'd put an end to that. She was going by what it says in the Bible: Spare the rod and spoil the child. She let Lee handle everything because he was the man of the house. Well, sometimes you have to put your foot down and be the woman of the house and I told her so too. If a man can't carry on like a man is supposed to, then a woman has to take over.

"Tim couldn't do anything to please him, even after he got grown. Lee was always scolding and mistreating him, up until a couple of years before he passed. I never understood why he mistreated Tim. It was just him, not their daughter."

"She let Lee handle everything because he was the man of the house. Well, sometimes you have to put your foot down and be the woman of the house and I told her so too."

I mention that Lee may have endured the same abuse from his parents. Evelyn retorts, "That don't mean you treat people that way. You are supposed to treat them better than you were treated!"

She does recognize some worthy traits in Lee. "We live on a farm about 30 miles away from Meridian. Whenever we were in the hospital there for anything, he would visit us every day and go out of his way to help us in any way, day or night. Also, if there was bad weather coming in, he would always call and warn us. 'There's a tornado or heavy rain coming, you better get in the house,' he'd say. And he provided good for his family."

Barclay's Aunt Shirley, his mom's youngest sister, is only four years older than Barclay. She played often at the Fryery home when she was young, with Barclay who was "a very typical little boy. I did not witness any abuse," she says. "I just know that his father was very stern and strict, as a lot of country dads were back then." I ask if Shirley ever saw Lee express pride in his son. "I did. When Tim had his TV shows, Lee was very proud of him. He always called and made sure we were watching. He was proud of his work and his success. I just think he could not accept what Tim had claimed to have become. He'd tell me, 'Dad does not accept me being gay or who I am.' I didn't hear any of those conversations, but I know there was bitterness between them.

"The relationship got off to a rough start after Tim moved back here. Tim was proud to be who he was, proud to be gay. In the South, you don't come home and announce that. People here live a quiet life. Tim does not have a filter; he wanted people to know and to accept, and people weren't ready. Lee did not want to talk about or digest it."

> *"Tim was proud to be who he was, proud to be gay. In the South, you don't come home and announce that."*

Barclay suggests I also get Susie's (Choo's) opinion of his father. "Overall, Lee was a good man," says Susie. "He was comical without trying to be comical, and because of that he earned the nickname 'Barney Fife,' though I'm not sure he was ever called that to his face. In spite of his comical ways, Lee was the man to go to if something needed to be taken care of. He knew how to get things done and was always glad to help. I have many, many memories of Lee, but there is one that stands out from the rest. Barclay had been invited to give a talk at the Riley Center here several years ago. I had the privilege of sitting with his parents, so I had a ringside seat. When Barclay finished, Lee stood up with tears in his eyes and began to clap. Seeing firsthand the pride he felt for his son melted my heart. I will never forget it."

Lee Fryery died on April 18, 2015, at the age of 82.

"I wrote a beautiful obituary," says Barclay. "His funeral was one of the most elegant ever. I planned every detail. The music was 18th-century Baroque: 'Water Music' by Handel, 'The Four Seasons' (Spring) by Vivaldi, and Handel's 'Hallelujah Chorus.' For flowers, I had only white Phalaenopsis orchids in urns on pedestals, along with a casket piece of giant branches and green leaves—it was very strong and masculine and most atypical. No one else has done it quite that way. It was a huge statement. No ugly funeral flowers were allowed. I called every florist in town and told them, if people called, it was this or nothing. My mother, sister, and I each laid a single white Polo rose on the casket as it was lowered into the ground. I did all this mainly because he always said that *real men* do not set the table at Christmas, much less design."

I asked Barclay if there was some satisfaction in getting the last word on that small-minded dictum? "Yes," he said. "I also wanted to make sure he was truly dead. It was absolutely my mission."

THE OTHER LAYERS OF THE SILVER lining to Barclay's return to Mississippi are less murky. "I've been able to spend time with my mother," says Barclay. "I helped Bug get through a terrible divorce. I made a lovely home for myself and my babies, Pooh and Princess, to deal with the cancer journey. I could not have done any of this in Greenwich quite the same way."

During the first year of that journey, Barclay did question if Mississippi was the right place to seek treatment. In June of 2015, he was misdiagnosed. "I had a swollen lymph node," explains Barclay. "They first told me it was a cold and then sent me home with penicillin. In November, my HIV doctor said, 'Oh no, something is wrong there. You've got to have it biopsied.' I was still not even thinking cancer, or, worse, death, doom, and gloom. I was in denial. I refused to even think I had cancer.

"My sister and Aunt Shirley were there on either side of me when I went in to have the biopsy done. Then I didn't think about it. I wasn't going to let that ruin my Christmas. In January, it hit me like a ton of bricks."

Barclay began posting his cancer saga on Facebook. "The only way I survived in a healthy mindset was by writing about it and sharing," says Barclay, who at the time, in the winter of 2016 was given seven months to live. "I was completely myself. I took criticism for that from people here in my hometown. I didn't let that bother me for long, because it's not their journey. It's my journey. I

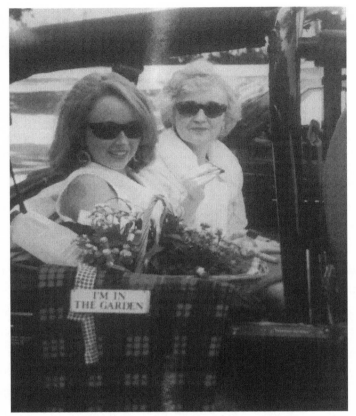

Barclay's sister and mom heading to a picnic organized by Barclay

have 10,000 friends, between subscribers and two Facebook pages. It affects a lot of lives. My posts are public, so it goes everywhere. That's why I blog on Facebook—it spreads faster." Barclay's writing therapy became more than that. His Facebook friends became part of the journey—they even influenced the itinerary.

> *"The only way I survived in a healthy mindset was by writing about it and sharing."*

"A person I'd been nice to at Starbucks in Greenwich years ago saw my posts and told me, 'Dr. Arlen will help you! He has a study. I'll make sure you are in it; he has a cure.' So that's what started my cancer journey. I flew to Greenwich and Bill Ford took me in. I still didn't think I was going to die. I was advertising to come and do a one-day design makeover of your home for $500. I really thought I could work through it.

"An angel came out of the woodwork, who I'd only met once: Ann Marenakos. She took me to radiation every day, bought me a sandwich to make sure I had food in my stomach, gave me a hug and kiss after each one. I mean who does that? Just a wonderful creature. So I had love surrounding me. I still thought I could beat it.

"I returned in July for surgery to remove the tumor in my neck. Leigh Cross—my favorite kitten, a true glamor-puss right here in Mississippi—paid my plane fare, which was $1,000! In Greenwich, I stayed with my friend, Elihys England, the countess. (She's a Hungarian countess. She doesn't walk around calling herself that, but I get a kick out of it, so I do.) I went to Versailles for lunch. They'd give me a discount. It was like advertising on the sidewalk. I bumped into all sorts of people and got all sorts of leads. Then I'm at the countess's house, and I'm pulling myself up the staircase to my guest suite and my left kidney is hurting. I think, *Oh no.* I lived with that for two weeks, then my energy started going.

> ## *"Dr. Arlen said with urgency in his voice: Go home, go back amongst your pretty things."*

"Dr. Arlen ordered cat scans and found lesions in my left kidney and on my spine. The cancer was in some lymph nodes, but they still couldn't find the mother, the primary source. At that point, Dr. Arlen said with urgency in his voice: 'Go home, go back amongst your pretty things, do a round of chemo and radiation. You'll be fine in two years.' So I packed up my Louis and came home a week early." Barclay notes that his Louis Vuitton suitcase, which he loves, has a broken zipper and holes in it. It was not something he could sell to pay his medical bills.

"I couldn't work, but I had to keep my head held high like Mother taught me. Like that little train: I think I can. No, not I think I can; I *know* I can." At one point in our interview, the TV suddenly turns on to *Thomas the Train*, tooting through his town. Barclay tells me he loves that show and PBS Kids. It must be just about as far away from the thought of cancer as you can get.

Barclay continues, "I thought, *I've survived before. I can survive cancer.*" He pauses for a long time before admitting, quietly, "It's got me this time. I can't escape anymore. Even with that, I have resolve."

"I thought, I've survived before. I can survive cancer."

There is another saying Barclay learned from his mom. It's embroidered on the throw pillow he likes the Angels to fluff before they leave each day. "Wrap it up," it reads. It means: get it done, move on with your life, don't wallow or dillydally.

But wrapping up a life . . . It's hard to wrap your mind around that.

Barclay has had friends from all over the globe offering to fly him to Germany or Paris for miracle treatments. However, Barclay has reached the stage of being realistic. It's time to wrap it up. "The doctors here had not been wrong," he says. "The cancer has metastasized; it's all over the place. There are blood clots all over my body.

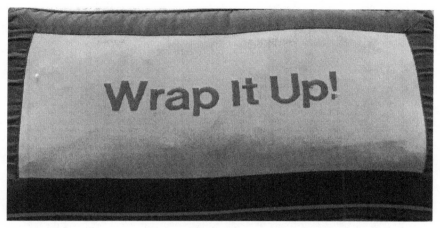

Barclay's decorator pillow, embroidered with one of his mom's favorite sayings

So they can't treat me, as they are afraid a clot will go straight to my head and kill me. All this fluid is from lymph drainage," Barclay explains, as he shows me how his hand has left an indentation just from resting on his leg. "My feet are scaling and bursting, they are so swollen." He winces in pain as he makes his way to the bathroom or the front door to receive friends.

While Barclay has come to terms with his prognosis, he'd rather not have the ugly side of cancer in his face. "I can't even look in the mirror," he says. "I can look shoulder up and fix my hair and make sure I'm presentable and clean. I wear my tartan blanket over my legs. I can't look at the changes that have happened. I know that's denial, but some of that denial helps you get through a period. It's a coping mechanism.

"I want to go to bed and not wake up, when it's meant to be. When I've done what I can do."

"It's a weird case. My cancer is immune-system related. It doesn't have any labels on it, and that's why it is so bizarre and changing all the time. It's in my kidney, joints, lymph nodes—all over my body, except from the chest up. And I pray every day: God have mercy, I don't want to lose my mind, my voice. I've got a nice voice, a nice mind; I want to communicate. I want to go to bed and not wake up, when it's meant to be. When I've done what I can do.

"Each night, I don't know if I'll wake up, but I go to bed, stretch out with Teddy and the Princess, and I go to sleep and forget that I'm sick. I have wonderful, beautiful dreams, filled with different people I know. Sometimes they don't make sense and I wake up and I say *wooooow*. I sit on the side of the bed and then I feel the pain in my legs, and I realize that I have what I have. I don't sit up and fret. I escape in my sleep. If I wake up, I write about it and make something positive out of it."

"Look at me, I mean I have cancer and I'm dying, but I had a wonderful life."

Looking back on his life, Barclay says, "Often you wonder if the stork dropped you in the wrong family. You really do. But my parents were very proud of me. Some children are touched, and I was touched and abused because of it. But look at me, I mean I have cancer and I'm dying, but I had a wonderful life. Insecurity-wise, it took me years to get over that, but I got over it. If you can't love yourself, you can't love anybody. Every one of the bullies from high school has seen my career, and they've all called and apologized. And of course I forgave them. That's what you do when someone asks sincerely." (One of them is a household name now, and Barclay has designed several homes for him.)

"Every time I hear someone criticizing someone else, I stop them," says Barclay. "I want to know who they are from my perspective. It's almost like when I walk into a house. I want to walk into it and feel inspired or see where I want to edit it."

The way to closure for Barclay is seizing every day, rather than counting how many days he has left.

Even on his deathbed—which sounds like such a misnomer when applied to the way Barclay is living his final chapter—Barclay is still editing rooms as well. Friends send him photos and he gives advice. Several projects await should "a miracle happen." The way to closure for Barclay is seizing every day, rather than counting how many days he has left.

His friend Karolina Hagman, a former Ford Model, sent him a remedy that he tried for the first time the morning of our interview. "She talked me into trying something else," he says, explaining that he and Karolina bonded in New York years ago, "through some horrible, snotty people. Well, they were not horrible, but compared to *her* they were! She is six feet tall and blonde. We escorted each other to parties and became like siblings. She calls me 'broder.'"

"Fear, uncertainly, doubt—they should be dirty words in cancer. I just try not to have them in my life. I push out sadness. I don't want sadness."

He directs me to, "Look in the fridge. There are two gallons, one for stress and one for cancer. They look and taste like water. It's a potion made by scientists in New Jersey. I took an ounce of each this morning. Never think that because I give up the ghost that I'm really giving up the ghost, because we are Leos, remember! Unless a miracle happens or God heals me or this potion works, I'm not getting my hopes up. But I'm staying positive. What do I have to lose? Fear, uncertainly, doubt—they should be dirty words in cancer. I just try not to have them in my life.

"I push out sadness. I don't want sadness. I wake up every day and I pray. Even when I thought I was an agnostic I did this. I prayed every day: help me be the very best person I can be, forgive me for any wrongdoings, help me make an impact. I prayed that every morning and every night before I went to sleep for my whole life. I think you should be the very best you can be, and sadness doesn't fit into that equation."

CHAPTER 7

After-Party and After-Life

Plans for an Ultra-Chic Life Celebration and Designs for Heaven

"LAST WEEK I PLANNED MY AFTER-party," Barclay tells me. "Renae has the whole menu. My sister can't wrap her head around that at all. She said, 'How can you wrap your head around that?' I told her, 'It's like a design project. You have this impossible house and you have to wrap your mind around it. Otherwise, you can't do it.'" It only makes sense that the man in Mississippi most capable of creating an ultra-classy event ought to plan it.

> *"It's like a design project. You have this impossible house and you have to wrap your mind around it."*

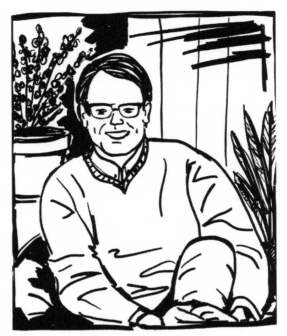

A portrait by Zoe Wodarz commissioned for this book, based on a photograph of Barclay in Chuck and Martha Baker's book, The Outdoor Living Room

"I was going to have it here," says Barclay, meaning the several hundred square feet we are sitting in. But considering how many friends he has, he realizes that would be like putting an enormous sleigh bed in Jordan Force's modest bedroom. Fortunately, Barclay knows all the right people.

"I called Kate and asked if we could have the main gallery and the entrance hall at the Museum of Art," he says. His Angel Kate granted his wish. "We are going to have this column with the David head," Barclay explains, switching into professional designer mode and gesturing toward the column in his bedroom. "We will have my sterling silver wine bucket fashioned into an urn, containing my ashes, in the middle of the main gallery. There's going to be this picture"— he points at the Leslie Mueller

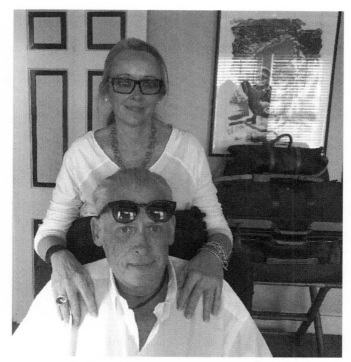

Barclay and "Bug," during my visit to Meridian on March 21, 2017

portrait of him and Mr. Pooh—"and possibly this wall, behind the urn and the column. They had discussed putting up all of my art. I advised we just display the art from my bedroom. The wall will include: antlers, coats of arms, portraits, architectural drawings, Greco Roman medallions, and more antlers—not unlike the Barnes Collection in Pennsylvania. They've photographed my room so they can recreate it.

"There will be a dress code: gray, black, or white, or you don't get in. Just like P. Diddy. There will be jazz, classical, opera, or Baroque 18th-century music from Pandora piped in.

"I'm famous for my afternoon coffees, making lattes with finger sandwiches and something sweet, so we are serving Starbuck's lattes, finger sandwiches, a sweet, and I'm throwing in a fabulous

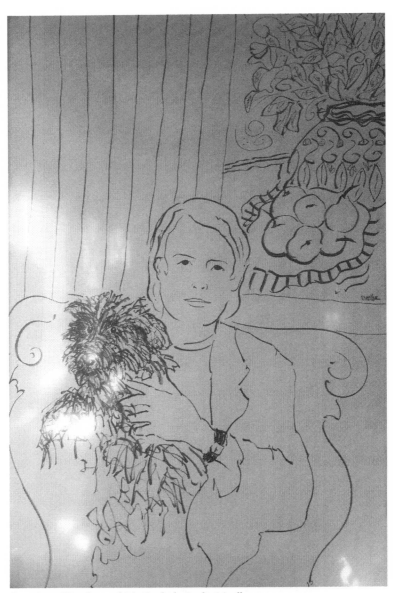

Drawing of Barclay and Mr. Pooh, by Leslie Mueller

dash of roasted Brussels sprouts sautéed in garlic and olive oil and sprinkled with parmesan—because they are my favorite since I've been sick and they are little cancer fighters. Cancer hates cabbage! And all of my old society ladies will come. My It girls will come. I used to have four society ladies with me in my living room on every other Sunday afternoon. And then my It girls, my kittens, would come to have coffee with me one-on-one. When I got cancer, it made that hard.

"The inspiration for that came from Daniel. He suggested, 'You let friends know that you are free between 3 and 5 on Sundays.' Southern women used to send out 'at-home cards.' My mother had them. The card gave a day and time range when they would be home to receive guests, as you didn't dare just drop in on people in the South and this way the host didn't need to plan a whole menu. You'd offer finger foods, sweets, cocktails depending on timing. I still use an at-home card if I'm having a casual party. I've kept it alive. That's my take on my after-party with the coffee and sandwiches. Your party can be anything you want, whatever your fantasy. I thought it would be nice to do something I was known for.

> *"Your party can be anything you want, whatever your fantasy."*

"The flowers will be in the center of the center table—as many white roses as we can afford, all cut Ralph-Lauren style, and white orchids, ferns, and moss. So the palette will be white and green only. No funeral flowers! Doesn't that sound festive and fabulous?

"I'm planning on 50 to 100 people. We'll do an invitation on Facebook and one to text to people—with a very modern design. I figure it should be five weeks out from the demise, because that way guests have no excuse not to be there. People will have time to get themselves organized. My friends who have never met each other will meet on that day. I want no sorrow, no sadness. I'll have my three angels, Renae, Kate, and Choo, say something positive about me. My sister will be too broken up."

"The palette will be white and green only. No funeral flowers! Doesn't that sound festive and fabulous?"

I look for signs of the marshmallow under the stoic front, but this Fryery is holding it together. Barclay still has a guest list to make, an invitation to design. He's following "Fluff" Tip #4: Get up and plan your day. He is not sitting around waiting for the end.

Barclay is not obsessing about death, but he also is not neglecting his what-if philosophy. "I've gotten more in touch with my religious self," he says. "I thought I was an agnostic all these years. But if there is a heaven, I want to decorate in heaven. I want to throw it around up there. I don't want to go to hell, if there is a hell. I prayed and got it all right. I'm not going to Bible thump, but you know, the what-if. I want to make sure that I am covered in all areas. What if someone comes for a visit? Your house is pulled together. What if . . . has been my entire life.

"I thought I was an agnostic all these years. But if there is a heaven, I want to decorate in heaven."

"A friend of mine, Andrea Ramsey, helped me accept Christ back into my life, so I go to heaven to make sure I can do her mansion up there! She is a prosecutor and her husband is a minister.

Her daughter Amicia, the TV reporter who did the HIV story, lives next door. She's quite beautiful and quite wonderful. She has light brown skin, so the landlord didn't want to rent to her. She asked me, 'What is she?'"

Knowing how to manage the southern mentality, Barclay responded, "French, probably Jewish."

She got the apartment. "Her mother and I became great friends," says Barclay. "I love the fact that an African American hardcore prosecutor would connect with the likes of me! She thought I was a snob at first. Now she calls me her 'brother from another mother,'" says Barclay. "She's hoping I can do her house in Illinois in July. If things don't go the way we hope, I'll do her place in heaven."

BARCLAY AND I HAVE TALKED ALL DAY. We talked through his usual 6 p.m. nap and through dinnertime, forgetting to eat. He doesn't have much of an appetite but he suggests I try the chicken pot pie a friend dropped for him. I pad into the kitchen in socks, having kicked off my shoes some hours ago. A place that was brand-new to me nine hours before now feels so familiar. I open the fridge, where the miracle potion sits amidst a bounty of nourishing gifts from the angels watching over Barclay. I move slowly as I turn on the oven, place the pie inside on the rack, and peruse the stack of pretty plates on the stovetop. I need to head back to Jackson, but I dread leaving.

Before today, Barclay and I knew each other on a work basis and from a few lunches. Now I feel like I've known him since he whizzed around on a red tricycle trying to impress his babysitter. I've seen his wounds—both buried ones he rarely reveals and the raw ones cancer has bestowed. The rich timbre of his voice has curled up in my ear for the day like Princess Royale sprawled in the sun. I've inhabited his home, wallpapered with mementos from his vibrant life, and tried to absorb every inch. For 20 minutes, I even nestled up on his bed, placing my head on his perfectly fluffed pillow, for a rest. The bed where he dreams beautiful dreams and forgets about the cancer. The bed where cancer may take him one day soon.

The aroma of the baking pie drifts into Barclay's bedroom. It smells like my Grammie's house when I was little, when life sprawled out endlessly before me.

"Do you think you have everything you need? Did you get what you want?" asks Barclay as I finish the comfort food I wish he could share with me.

"Oh, my goodness," I respond, "I have so much more than I anticipated." I label six voice record files as Barclay 1 through 6, and the enormity of the job ahead hits. I need him to be here to help me see this project through, to run this mad dash with me and cross the finish line, holding this book in his hands. But, what if? . . . We are facing the worst kind of deadline possible.

I'm stoic, just like Barclay, but a lump forms in my throat as I begin packing up my bag. All the pretty things around us make this better than a hospital farewell, but the portraits and pillows go blurry as the tears I'm trying to hold back slip out. Barclay remains strong. He pulls himself up from his seat and we embrace. I utter, "I don't want to say good-bye."

"Don't ever say good-bye. Just say: I'll see you when I see you."

"No, no," says Barclay. "Don't ever say good-bye. Just say: I'll see you when I see you."

"I'll see you when I see you, Barclay."

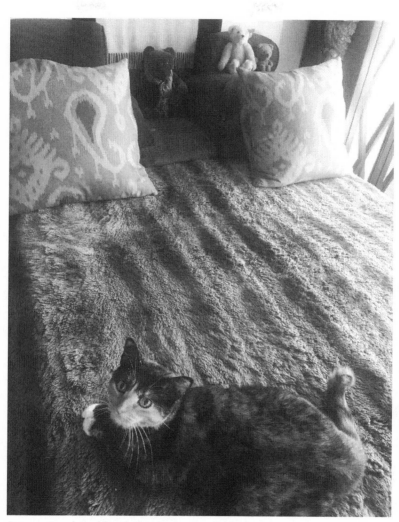

Princess Royale and Barclay's teddy bears on his bed

Epilogue

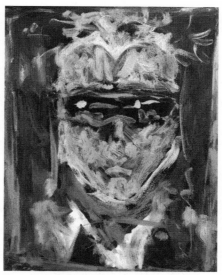

"Super Hero Barclay," painted by Terry Cherry in April of 2017

TWO MONTHS HAVE PASSED SINCE I spent the day interviewing Barclay in Meridian. The time has been measured in word counts and chapters, worsening symptoms and I-love-yous. I've learned you always say "I love you" when it might be the last time you hear a friend's voice. I've learned that "friend" is an inadequate term for a co-author whose life you are immersed in, especially when that life has reached its most fragile moment.

Soon after my arrival back in Connecticut, I began to count on my dawn text greeting from Barclay—"Good morning, sunshine . . . Good mornya!"—reassuring me that my partner was still out there. It became a reflex for me each morning to reach over to my nightstand, pick up my phone, read Barclay's message, and sigh with relief. Sometimes I received a bonus singing voice mail. I continue to listen to them whenever I'm down and my heart needs a kick start.

Barclay and I developed a routine this spring. After his cheery early salute to the day and his daily Facebook greeting to the world, we got to work. I transcribed the interviews and dove into writing, knowing I didn't have time to ponder, outline, or obsess about perfection. My four kids' busy lives were background chatter to the voice that dominated my days: Barclay's voice. I heard it directly by phone, several times a day at least, and via the steady pings of text and Facebook messages that came in as late as 1:30 a.m., as early as 4:30 a.m.

But most of all, Barclay's voice came to me as I wrote. It flowed into my head and onto the page with ease. I wrote on bleachers at ball fields, in waiting rooms at doctor's offices, during middle school transition meetings, and mostly late at night when the kids were in bed. Barclay would be awake from his evening nap then, and we'd consult on facts and name spellings, cover photos and book formats. I could feel the project fueling him, reviving his zest for life, despite constant pain. I encouraged him, "Hang in there. I need you!" He texted back, "You are giving me the strength to carry on. Thank you. I will not let you down. I haven't felt this alive since before the recession."

For the first month of our prolific work, I could hear the power in Barclay's voice growing. I wondered if the magic potion of words might be more effective than the liquid form in his fridge. Barclay's enthusiasm served as the engine for our endeavor, and he lived for our readings . . . literally.

When I read him the prologue, I was nervous about whether he would like it, whether I had come anywhere close to capturing in a few pages the turmoil of the last two years of his life. I worried it would upset him. When I got to the section in which I repeated his Facebook announcement of his terminal diagnosis and treatment dead-end, my voice grew shaky. When writing, I found the detachment I needed to stay focused; reading, my throat tightened and the pent-up tears trickled out. I heard mostly an eerie silence on the other end as I read, and then, as I finished, gentle sobbing.

After a few moments, I asked, "Are you okay?"

I could hear Barclay crying. In almost a whisper, he said, "It's beautiful, Jill. Beautiful. It's perfect. Thank you."

I realized this was why I was writing—for Barclay first, for those who would learn from his wisdom or be fascinated by his life second. I just needed him to feel this way about every chapter and my job was done.

From then on, I tried to keep pace with Barclay's frequent requests: "Can we read today? . . . Are we reading tonight? . . . Is the next chapter finished?" Laundry and dishes piled up. The kids got used to me telling them that right now Barclay needed me more than they did. He likened the book to a series of "fireside chats with Barclay." He loved it.

As the weeks passed and Barclay and I became deeply bonded by the project and his circumstances, our efforts—whether we were writing, or marketing on Facebook—became seamless. "We are speaking in one voice," Barclay told me. I also found myself being friendlier to gas station attendants and grocery baggers and strangers on the street, bestowing smiles and spreading kindness as Barclay would.

AS I WAS WRITING "CLOSURE," I realized I'd missed an important question—or perhaps I'd been too shy to ask back before I knew almost everything about Barclay.

"Did you have any great loves?" I asked him during a phone call.

"My work and me. My friends. The world. Travel. Paris. No men," he replied.

"None?"

"I had loves but no great love. Women always found me more attractive than men," explained Barclay. "I did not fit the typical gay mold of what they were looking for. I was looking for the finest things in life—the finest clothes, the finest neighborhood to live in, the finest furnishings. And so I went for extraordinary men from the first families of the US, Europe, the Middle East. Duponts, Rockefellers—I dated them. Men like that live off inheritances and don't work. They drank. They did drugs. I dated viscounts in London and princes from Saudi Arabia, Iran, and France. My career got in the way, and their families got in the way. They had to marry the right girl and have a certain number of children. I wasn't looking to meet someone, move in together and bring my furniture. I like my own space."

He admitted that Oscar Larrat was a love. "He was half marquis, the grandson of a king and a maid. He came to America and I fell madly in love," recalled Barclay. "I dated other upper-class boys, chevalier boys; the coat-of-arms ring on their pinky tells you they're upper class. They would see how I was dressed, how I carried myself. I never sought them out. They came to me. Phillip of Austria was one. He is half prince—his grandmother was a Hapsburg—and half train conductor.

"All the possible great loves became best friends. Oscar was one. Phillip of Austria another. Daniel was another. That way I would not lose them. We had brief relationships, but I didn't want to mess with the friendships and break up and be nasty and all that. David Gruning, a doctor's son from Fairfield, Connecticut, was my first long relationship. When I got HIV, he left. My next boyfriend, Carlos Barrios, a pop star, left when I lost my money. You don't do that! That's when I spiraled into depression.

"The most fulfilling relationships I've had in my life were with women. I consider them wives and girlfriends; we just don't have sex, which really is only 3 percent of the formula for a good relationship. I'm just more compatible with women. They are more compassionate. I can't stand most men; I think because of the way my father treated me. It took years for me to get over that and find a way to love myself. Most men don't love themselves."

I wondered if it made Barclay sad, to not have found love.

"Oh no," he said without hesitation. "I had my career and my babies. I had my friends."

MAYBE ONLY SOMEONE WHO DID not pour his heart into one mate could nurture the love fest that I witnessed in Barclay's life over the last couple of months. Whenever he was touched by a kind gesture or moving comment, he called and shared the details with me. On Easter, in mid-April, Barclay received 45 handmade Easter cards from students at PS 11 elementary school in Manhattan. They were sent anonymously, arranged by one of the many friends and fans who brightened Barclay's days in small and big ways. Barclay responded with a goofy selfie on Facebook of himself disguised as the Easter Bunny. At moments like that, I thought, *Maybe he will pull through. Maybe there will be a miracle.*

> "*When you do things from your soul, you feel a river moving in you, a joy.*
> —Rumi" (Facebook Post, May 3, 2017)

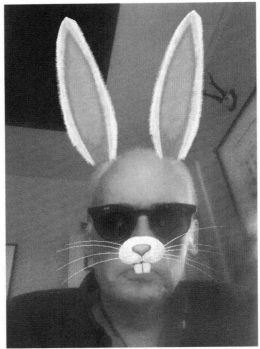

Barclay's Facebook post on Easter 2017

We made it to May. Barclay told me he now maneuvered around his apartment with the aid of his "Range Rovero." That was his chic translation for *steel gray walker.* He continued to spend 10 hours a day sitting in his chair, but it was not idle time. One day he messaged me to tell me: "I just had a spontaneous luncheon in my bedroom with my hippie rocker hairdresser Jessica; my Aunt Shirley, a preppy RN nurse; and Kate Cherry, the director of the Meridian Museum of Art—four people who normally would not speak to each other, much less nosh together. We had authentic tacos à la East LA from a Mexican food truck. Everyone had a blast listening to Parisian trip hop world music. It was marvelous!"

Barclay posed for another portrait, painted by Kate's husband, to add to his collection and to the book. "Needless to say, I have been an avid art collector since age 22," he wrote on Facebook. "Terry Cherry, art professor extraordinaire, recently finished a commissioned portrait of Your Barclay for my new book, *Cancer Looks Good on You*, and I simply adore it. It's entitled Super Hero Barclay! It is a reverse painting on glass, a French technique called Verre Eglomise! Terry had intended on painting me wearing my trademark Paul Smith tortoise horn rims, but somehow it turned out looking like a character from a Marvel comic. Since my eyes are so prominent, the eyeglasses become a mask instead . . . very interesting! Or am I a patron at the Venice Carnival or is it simply a death mask . . ."

On May 5, I didn't hear from Barclay for six hours. No pings, no calls, no Facebook posts. This made me uneasy because Barclay never went MIA for that long. At 4 p.m. he called me via Facebook, sounding more chipper than ever. "Where have you been?" I scolded like an anxious mother.

"I've been doing a design job!" he said excitedly. "I did Karen and Sonny Rush's house, of Rush Foundation Hospital. I did it right here from my chair, using floor plans and photos. It's a three-story townhouse in Oxford, Mississippi, where I went to school. I came right to life. Never for a second was I tired. I went very Hollywood, with navy blue double front doors, light gray painted brick, and white high-gloss shutters—the reverse of what you'd usually do. It's going to be absolutely glamorous, the best house in town by far."

Karen, a friend of Barclay's, had been out of touch. Barclay said, "She told me, 'I'm so sorry we weren't together this whole time.' I replied, 'We weren't meant to be. We are meant to reconnect now, and I'll be in heaven, waiting to do your house there.'" Karen made the reality of bills in this life a little easier for Barclay by buying his Hermes scarf. He was so tickled about his prosperous and rewarding day.

Susie later told me, "Barclay didn't want to let on how much trouble he was having with his vision at this point. He wasn't able to see well enough to draw out the design, so he enlisted me to do that part. It was like taking dictation in the form of art, with many changes over a couple days until we finally got it. He really perked up during that time and for that little while, the cancer was forgotten."

Soon after that, Barclay received a message from a friend who comes from one of "the top families in the world." She wrote: "I will confide to you that I was suicidal last week. Things have been rough financially and therefore emotionally. I began planning my exit and then, you came into my mind. You saved my life by being the example of how precious life is. How I should not throw it away when you are fighting every day. Thank you, my friend."

ON MAY 8TH, BARCLAY TOOK a turn for the worse. "The neuro-pathy is moving up my body," he told me, his voice weak and hoarse. "It's affecting my fingertips. I can't type." My stomach dropped, thinking of him rendered mute in his Facebook sanctuary. He promised to send me a box of magazines, his cherished sketchbook, and photos to use for the interior of the book. He insisted he send them that very day.

That afternoon Barclay texted me: "Can we read some of the book now?"

I was working on "Closure," but it wasn't quite done and I had to shuttle kids around for several hours. So I wrote, "I'd like to get the chapter finished first. Tomorrow for sure!"

He responded, "First of all, I love you, but I, especially, am not always promised a tomorrow. I am very ill today, out of the blue. Please try and seize the day."

Panic settled in my heart then and would stay for the duration of this journey.

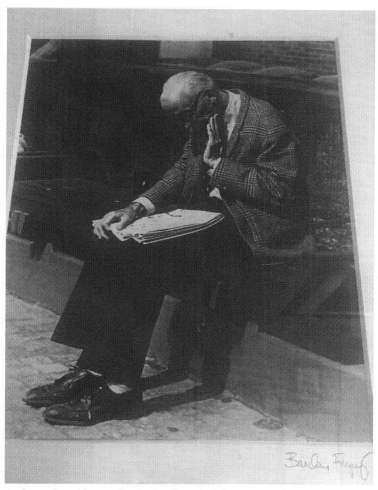

A photo of an old man, shot by Barclay, which hangs in his kitchen

Of course I called Barclay. His voice was almost completely gone. I read what I had so far in the chapter, but it felt unfinished. Unfinished like the life of a 56-year-old being robbed of the three more decades he deserved.

I wrote faster. When I heard the song about Alexander Hamilton writing like he was running out of time, I knew the feeling. A friend of mine began building a website for the book, where people would be able to pre-order. They needed to show their support NOW. I know Leos. Barclay wanted the adoration. He wanted to share his story and be heard. He deserved it. It was on me to make it happen.

We raced to finalize a cover concept, to secure the original photo from a couple who also has four kids. They were busy with shoots during the day and tucking in their children at night and . . . they could get us the photo "in two weeks." No, no, no! "Barclay may not have two weeks!" I bellowed into the phone. The photo landed in my inbox the next morning.

I asked Barclay what shade of pink he wanted as a pop of color on the cover. He said it should be "the pink from a bullfighter's stocking in Spain or the South of France. That's the pink on my low-slung Parsons bench fashioned into a TV stand in my bedroom. I saw a bullfight and didn't like the suffering, but I saw those pink stockings and had to run out and find fabric in that shade!" That is so like Barclay, to find beauty on a backdrop of pain.

The website was coming together, but the e-commerce setup was complex and time consuming. Barclay's morphine dosage increased. His vision worsened. He was seeing double. Triple. His Facebook messages became garbled. He wanted to see the site, while he could still see at all, but it wasn't ready yet. My friend was scrambling. "I don't know how much time he has," I said, my stomach winding into macramé knots.

What if he can't see it? What if that beautiful cover photo of breathtakingly handsome Barclay goes live and it's too late? All this time we've been striving to have the book in his hands before he goes. But now that goal feels like it is slipping away. And I can't imagine holding the book in my hands without my co-author here to share the celebration.

On Saturday, May 13th, Barclay sounded better. He was like a racehorse at the starting gate, desperate to share the website and watch the book take off. We planned a soft launch on Sunday but technicalities interfered. We needed to delay until Monday morning. Barclay was disappointed but put on a positive front. "I understand," he said. He was always patient and understanding, though the ticking of the clock must have been deafening in his head.

On Sunday evening, he texted, "Very ill." I called him and he sounded horrible. "Can you read the last chapter?" he asked weakly. I had just finished it that day. I began reading, with Barclay wheezing on the other end of the line. I read as fast as I could get the words out.

On Monday, May 15th, I woke up and saw no morning text from Barclay. I tried not to panic. I checked Facebook. At 3:43 a.m., he had posted: "Good morning world! Happy Monday! Have a Super Day!" At 5:19 a.m., he had shared a video about Paris. Then nothing. I typed in cancerlooksgoodonyou.com and saw that we were ready to share our book with the world. I called Barclay. No answer. I messaged him. No answer. I texted him. No answer.

Deflated, I announced the site on my Facebook page. My friends did not seem to share the zest for all-things-Barclay that his friends exhibit. I posted it to Barclay's page, but that hardly had the same standing-ovation effect that Barclay's own posts have on his audience.

Still nothing from Barclay. I realized that I probably needed to ask him for his Facebook password so that I could let his fans know about the book if he couldn't. It's one of those wrap-it-up details I hadn't thought of, because book writing enabled denial by precluding time for pondering what was ahead, beyond the completion of the project at hand. What if I was too late?

I texted Barclay and asked for his Facebook login and password, "for future reference, to cover what-ifs so I can keep the book and foundation alive there." Barclay envisioned a charity, the Barclay Fryery Foundation (I loved that the abbreviation for that is BFF), focused on teen suicide prevention and supporting LGBTQ youth. He had selected a board—many of them the angels from this book—which he had announced on Facebook. They applauded his idea and promised to fulfill Barclay's wishes. One member, who had been desperately depressed only recently, wrote: "Honored! Humbled. Once I find a way to express what this means to me/ what you mean to me I will write a proper declaration. For now please accept my pledge that your legacy will live on. You beautiful, priceless, generous, inspiring, heroic, perfect creature. I love you!"

Barclay understands *what-ifs*. My phone rang. Barclay! "I'm so glad to hear from you," I said, giddily. "Are you okay?"

I heard labored breathing on the other end and a thin whisper: "I'm very sick. All of my organs feel like lead." A chill went through my body. I had to ask him to repeat himself several times to understand what he said next: "I'm sending the passwords."

"Is someone there to help you, Barclay?"

I heard a faint "Yes . . . coming."

"I love you, Barclay. Please rest and get better. I will spread the word about the book!"

A gloom fell over me in my helplessness. I half-heartedly continued to share news of our book project.

Later that afternoon, Barclay called me. His voice was still gone and he was sick but he wanted to know how many orders we had. Earlier he had not had the energy to care, and I hardly could care without him in it with me. I dared to hope we had more time as a team. I offered to read him the book in its entirety, as I had been adding and editing since our chapter readings. It took several hours, during which I kept asking, "Should I go on?" He was groggy but always responded, "Yes, please."

At 2 a.m. that night, Barclay wrote, "Where do I find the link tomorrow morning so I can start marketing?"

Game on!

At 4:42 a.m., he sent me a tribute from Jane Coco Cowles, who had been ever-present cheering us on and had offered to help with book marketing: "You are an inspiration to me and forever will be. You see beauty in the ordinary, find humor in trying times, and show enduring strength amidst challenges. You follow your dreams and face your fears with dignity and grace. Watching you these last few months shows me that anything is possible when you love yourself and believe love endures even in darkness."

On Tuesday, Barclay began to reassert his presence in the Facebook world. The happy pings from my phone and laptop sprang back to life. He shared the link and orders started to flow in, each bolstering his will to live. I opened the box of photos and magazines he had sent. I chuckled to see that he had shipped the photos still in their heavy frames. On the day he'd prepared that box, he'd felt so ill that the urgency of getting the box to me had overrideen practicality. When I removed the bubble wrap from the photos, I smelled Barclay's apartment—the lavender and smoky tinge of the Marlboro Reds Barclay would sneak and didn't want me to write about. But I know he'd support me in telling youth: Cancer sticks are a Don't. Tobacco and all, the box—both a treasure chest and a tomb—overpowered me with emotion.

That evening Barclay sounded hoarse but reenergized. "I called Susan Frazier this morning, remember, the minister's daughter? We laughed and laughed," he said. Then he told me that he had ordered a pair of size-14 Gucci loafers—a treat for Barclay, who had given away much of the decadent wardrobe he'd had custom made

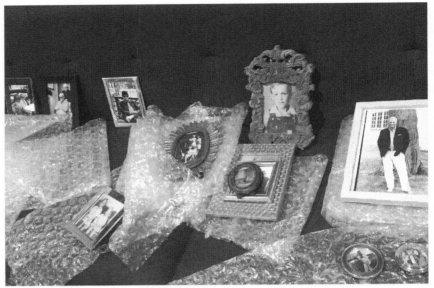

Barclay's cherished family photos spread across my couch

by Bernard the tailor in Paris. "I found them on eBay on sale, for a steal! They are 1953 style with a red and green stripe. My feet are too swollen to fit into my 13s. And what if I get on a talk show? I need to be ready!"

Oh my, I love this man. He must have learned early: when you get kicked to the ground, you gotta get right back up.

"My legs are spraying like a sprinkler from water retention," he said. I couldn't help but giggle at the image—and compliment him for his unwavering way with words. He added, "I feel like Mr. Green Jeans from the waist up and Lulu from *Hee Haw* from the waist down!"

Five more days have passed since then. Several of them have been excruciating for Barclay. He has lost strength in his legs and is falling down often as he tries to make it to the kitchen or bathroom. He admitted to me that pragmatism won out, and he did not actually buy the Gucci loafers. But his sense of humor has not failed.

"Last night I was stuck in my chair at 2 a.m.," he reported to me today. "I called the hospice company and they sent over this big, black woman, wearing a low-cut blouse. She lifted me with my face right in her abundant breasts and dragged me like that to the bed. It was the first time I ever motorboated with a woman!" We both had a good laugh about that.

For now, Barclay's beautiful voice is back. We hope to do some audio recordings and add them to the site. There are videos there as well, including "Meet Barclay, with Tommy Hilfiger," which captures Barclay's style, humor, and magnetism better than words ever could.

Please visit the site for updates on Barclay: **CancerLooksGood onYou.com**. I hope with all my heart that what you will see there is a photo of my dear Barclay, with this book in his hands.

Acknowledgments

ONLY DAYS AFTER BARCLAY ANNOUNCED that he had two weeks to two months to live, I had an epiphany. *We have to do a book*, I thought. It was a crazy idea, considering the timeline for potentially losing my co-author and the fact that I knew I couldn't do it without him. But Barclay loved the idea, and I had faith that he would outlive his doctors' prognosis—especially if he had this project fueling him. So the first person I want to thank, with all my heart, is the heart of this book: Barclay. Thank you for your passion, your wisdom, your willingness to share everything, and your belief in me to get this right. Thank you for being "on" 24 hours a day—eagerly helping in any way you could and sharing your infectious energy— when you must have felt so off. Thank you for holding on until the very last word was written. I only wish we could write ten more books together.

Barclay and I would both like to thank the Angels, Susie Womack Cannon ("Choo"), Kate Cherry, and Renae Gardner, who made this project possible by keeping Barclay's body and soul nourished and his practical and emotional needs met every step of the way. To Barclay's dear sister: He wanted a whole chapter devoted to you, Lisa. It was only my book structure issues that got in the way. Jane Coco Cowles and Elizabeth Guzman, our marketing angels—thank you! To every friend, family member, and fan quoted or mentioned in this book—and so many more who would have been, if we'd had more time—thank you for being there for Barclay.

To Yoonsun Lee, you earned your angel wings by passionately devoting your precious time to developing our cover concept and creating our gorgeous website: CancerLooksGoodonYou.com. To Brooke, Krissa, and Tabitha at Brooke Warner Coaching, thank you for your guidance, expertise, creative genius, and willingness to race frantically to the finish line with us. The results are beautiful.

Finally, I am so grateful to my husband, Ben, and my four kids, who loaned out their wife/mom for two months while her heart and mind were with Barclay.

About the Authors

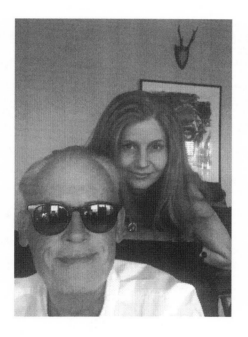

Jill Johnson

Jill Johnson is a freelance writer, founder of Modelingmentor.com/blog, and former editor-in-chief of *Tear Sheet* magazine, which she launched during her decade-long career as a fashion model. She has interviewed fashion icons (Lauren Hutton, Patrick Demarchelier, Heidi Klum, John Sahag, among many others), TV journalists

(Lara Spencer, Scott Pelley), and Broadway's best. She has covered all things catwalk and heavier topics, including infertility, eating disorders, autism, and education reform. She hopes to wrap up her modeling memoir soon, if she can get some time off from her part-time gig as her kids' chauffeur and laundress. Jill lives in Connecticut with her husband and four children, in a messy house by the beach. In her free time, she loves theatre, belly dancing (yes, you read that correctly), tap dancing, yoga, skiing, and horse riding.

BARCLAY FRYERY

Barclay Fryery is a renowned interior designer, TV personality, writer, and lifestyle coach. His work has been featured in *Elle Decor* and *House Beautiful*; on *House Wars*, the Style Network, and A&E; and his "Ask Barclay" column appeared in the *Greenwich Post* for 10 years. Over the last two years, Barclay has blogged about his cancer journey on Facebook and spread his philosophy of facing illness with grace and style. He promotes inclusivity and teaches his friends and fans to seize every day, no matter what challenges life presents. Barclay lives in Meridian, Mississippi, in a tidy apartment with his cat, Princess Royale. He enjoys classical music, art, theatre, lattes, and composing silly voice-mail songs.

Made in the USA
Middletown, DE
15 June 2018